*Extended Massive Orgasm*

*We would like to dedicate this book*
*to all students and pioneers of Sensuality*

## Contact Information

If you'd like more information on EMO and our courses,
please visit our website at www.extendedmassiveorgasm.com
or e-mail us at verasteve@aol.com.

## Ordering

Trade bookstores in the U.S. and Canada, please contact:

> Publishers Group West
> 1700 Fourth Street, Berkeley CA 94710
> Phone: (800) 788-3123    Fax: (510) 528-3444

Hunter House books are available at bulk discounts for textbook course adoptions;
to qualifying community, health care, and government organizations; and for special
promotions and fund-raising. For details please contact:

> Special Sales Department
> Hunter House Inc., PO Box 2914, Alameda CA 94501-0914
> Phone: (510) 865-5282    Fax: (510) 865-4295
> E-mail: ordering@hunterhouse.com

Individuals can order our books from most bookstores or by calling toll-free:
**(800) 266-5592**

# Extended Massive Orgasm

## How You Can Give and Receive Intense Sexual Pleasure

Steve Bodansky, Ph.D.
and Vera Bodansky, Ph.D.

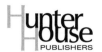

Hunter House PUBLISHERS

Hunter House Inc., Publishers
PO Box 2914
Alameda, CA 94501-0914


**Library of Congress Cataloging-in-Publication Data**
Bodansky, Steve.
    Extended massive orgasm : how you can give and receive intense sexual pleasure /
    Steve Bodansky and Vera Bodansky.
        p.cm.
    Includes bibliographical references and index.
    ISBN 0-89793-289-7 (paper)
            1. Sexual excitement.  2. Orgasm.  3. Sex instruction.  I. Bodansky, Vera.
II. Title.

HQ31 .B593 2000
613.9'6—dc21                                                                00-063146


**Project Credits**

COVER DESIGN: Madeleine Budnick

INTERIOR PHOTOGRAPHS: Ariel Parker

DEVELOPMENTAL EDITOR: Jeff Campbell

PROOFREADER: Michelle Ho

ILLUSTRATOR: Terri Sugg

GRAPHICS COORDINATOR: Ariel Parker

ASSOCIATE EDITOR: Alexandra Mummery

MARKETING ASSISTANT: Earlita Chenault

CUSTOMER SERVICE MANAGER: Christina Sverdrup

PUBLISHER: Kiran S. Rana

BOOK PRODUCTION: Brian Dittmar

MODELS: Erik Getman and Jessy Clark

LINE AND COPY EDITOR: Laura Harger

INDEXER: Kathy Talley-Jones

PRODUCTION MANAGER: Keri Northcott

ACQUISITIONS EDITOR: Jeanne Brondino

PUBLICITY MANAGER: Sarah Frederick

ORDER FULFILLMENT: Joel Irons

Printed and Bound by Publishers Press, Salt Lake City, UT
Manufactured in the United States of America

9  8  7  6  5  4  3            First Edition            02  03  04

# Table of Contents

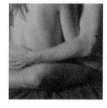

❧

# Acknowledgments

We are deeply grateful to Vic Baranco for five reasons. We are thankful that he created a place and an environment where sensuality could be studied and researched. We are doubly grateful that we were able to find each other and develop a relationship far greater than we could have hoped for. We are triply grateful for the information and techniques that we were able to learn from him. We are extremely thankful that he has generously allowed us and others to disseminate and pass on our versions of this information and techniques to our students. We are grateful to him and Diana Goens for having performed the first demonstration of an extended massive orgasm.

We also are grateful to Suzie Baranco who inspired and helped create the "More" philosophy.

We are grateful to our fellow pioneers who have helped so many learn about having wonderful sex lives. These include Brian Shekeloff, Alec Van Sinderen, Jackie Van Sinderen, Chris Anderson, Conway Anderson, Joe Hillis, Dica Hillis, Mark Scheur, Janet Scheur, Cindy Baranco, Diane Klass, Bob Klass, Marty Pearlstein, Dave Pettus, Bob Kerr, Marilyn Mohr, Judi Corey, Lori Hyland, Dick Hyland, Vicki Potts, Tracy St. John, and Robin Roberts.

We are indebted to Earl M. Marsh for introducing Vera to sensuality, Vic Baranco, and many other wonderful things.

We are fondly appreciative of Teri Sugg for creating such lovely drawings.

We are thankful to John Bussey for his encouragement and support.

We are grateful to Bruce and Regena Thomashauer of Relationship Technologies for their friendship and support.

We would like to thank Sandy Karp and Victor Kiernan for their help with the illustrations.

It has been a pleasure dealing with the staff at Hunter House Publishers, especially Jeanne Brondino, Kiran S. Rana, and Alexandra Mummery. Our heartfelt appreciation to Laura Harger for her tough job of turning our manuscript into something readable.

A final thanks to Steve's parents, Carl and Alice Bodansky, who although they did not always necessarily like what he was doing, nevertheless continued to love and lend their support.

## *Important Note*

The material in this book is intended to provide a review of information regarding extended massive orgasm. Every effort has been made to provide accurate and dependable information and the contents of this book have been compiled through professional research and in consultation with medical professionals. We believe that the sensuality advice given in this book poses no risk to any healthy person. However, if you have any genital infections, such as herpes, we recommend consulting your doctor before using this book.

The author, publisher, editors, and professionals quoted in the book cannot be held responsible for any error, omission, or dated material in the book. The author and publisher are not liable for any damage or injury or other adverse outcome of applying the information in this book. If you have questions concerning the application of the information described in this book, consult a qualified professional.

# *Introduction*

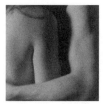

Vera and I met in May 1979 on a road named "Here" in an experimental university in northern California. My first words to Vera were, "My name is Steve, and I'd love to do you." To "do" someone or the act of "doing" is our own jargon for giving someone an orgasm by manual stimulation of their genitals. I had never used that line before and never used it again—I don't recommend it, but it did seem to work, and we were having "do" dates shortly thereafter.

The times were more open sexually in the 1970s than they are now, especially in California, and our community was very open sexually and even gave courses in sensuality. We were students at More University, which grew out of the "More" community. This community began in 1968 and still exists (although we're no longer members). Its founders believed that in order for a large group of people to successfully live close together and be intimate, they would have to handle sex. There were two ways that this could be done: either total celibacy, as with monks and nuns, or a high degree of structured openness and honesty between consenting adults. Because this was California in the 1970s, the second option was clearly preferable.

Vera and I did a lot of research together. We both majored in sensuality at More University, taking courses in Alternate Life Styles and Communication. We specifically researched the female orgasm and eventually received doctorates from More. Our work included all kinds of classes, mostly in techniques of "doing" and communication. (We are not sure when the word *doing* came to mean only manual stimulation in our work, but we continue to give the word this meaning today.) We were married in 1983, the third time for each of us. It's been more than twenty years since we met, and I still love doing Vera.

The information in this book is a combination of what we learned as students at More and what we have learned from our later careers as teachers, focusing upon sensuality, man/woman relationships, and communication. We taught first at More but later worked on our own, training teachers working in San Francisco and then working together as teachers. Specifically, this book is about extended massive orgasm (EMO), a technique that we have studied and taught for many years.

According to the leading sex therapists of the 1950s and 1960s (Kinsey, Masters, and Johnson), female orgasm constitutes, on average, nine to twelve contractions and lasts a few seconds after a long arousal period. Male orgasms are even shorter. Some women are able to have what are called multiple orgasms, which are a series of these small orgasms. But in our studies, Vera learned to have extended massive orgasms in each encounter, and I learned how to perform this magnificent act.

An EMO can last anywhere from a couple of minutes to three hours (that was enough for us) to even longer periods of time. An EMO is much more intense than the ordinary orgasm of nine to twelve contractions. An EMO can begin with or even before the first stroke, and it lasts as long as you like. EMOs are best and most efficiently produced with your hands. In this book, we give many techniques and examples of where and how to touch someone to produce the best orgasm.

One of our most informative courses is a demonstration of an extended massive orgasm, called the DEMO for short. The woman is naked on a special table in the front of the room, while the man, sitting on a stool next to her, stimulates her genitals. The man is fully clothed, and the experience is not in the least pornographic. The orgasm lasts for one hour; it is quite clinical yet still very intense and pleasurable, and affection is shown between the demonstrators. They are able to talk and answer questions while the orgasm happens. Additional information about EMO is presented before and after the demonstration.

This book has been written in the hope that more people will be able to add the pleasure of EMOs to their lives. First things first, though. In order to have a great sex life, you have to understand the similarities and differences between the behavior and thinking of both sexes. You also have to develop superior communication skills. This book includes information on both these topics as well as specific sexual techniques for producing EMOs.

Although this book focuses mostly on the female orgasm, this is a book for both women and men. Our goal is to teach women and men about having bigger and better orgasms and to teach lovers to be heroes by learning how to produce an EMO. Most of the techniques we describe for expanding her orgasm can be used to expand his as well. We also include some specific techniques for creating pleasure in a male body.

We usually teach this sensual information to heterosexuals, both singles and couples, but we've had some gay and lesbian students in the past, and they were able to expand their pleasure as well. This book can be read by both couples and singles, and couples can read it either together or alone. This book is also intended for both experts and novices—it can benefit people who are just beginning their sensual exploration as well as advanced students and even people who hope to teach sensuality.

"Doing" really begins with seducing and romancing a person's mind. Before touching someone's body, you have to touch his or her mind. If you are not able to do that, you will never be able to give your lover that special pleasure, no matter how well you can touch. Doing someone's mind really begins with focusing your total attention on that person. Noticing where they are at mentally and emotionally and how they respond to your attention allows you to proceed in your seduction. Of course, confidence in knowing that you can touch wonderfully is an asset, especially if it is quiet confidence, not egomaniacal bragging.

Learning to have EMOs is not as simple as some people might hope, but it's not as difficult as one might fear. A key lesson is the importance of the clitoris. Many men, including myself, are or were ignorant about the role of the clitoris. It's not that we did not want to know; we just had no idea. Before Masters and Johnson and Kinsey did their research, it was thought (at least in Western culture) that the vagina was the source of female orgasm and that the clitoris played a secondary role. I was married for the first time when I was twenty and was with my first wife for five years. She never mentioned the clitoris, nor did I hear it mentioned elsewhere. We did not talk about sex, and I have no idea if she had orgasms or even knew where her clitoris was. I wish we had had a "How to Do" book when we got married.

Since the sexual revolution and women's liberation movement, more people have become aware of female orgasm and the importance of the clitoris. Unfortunately, most people still do not know how to have a great orgasm every time they have sex, nor do they know how to produce one for their partners at will.

## How to Use This Book

In this book, you will learn about the most sensitive areas on your own body and on the bodies of the other sex. You'll learn the best ways and techniques to touch those areas to intensify sensation, and you'll learn how to keep an orgasm going. If your orgasm lasts just a few seconds now, it can expand to a few minutes. And once your orgasm lasts minutes, there is no reason you can't train to make it last indefinitely.

To become good at anything usually takes practice, so we don't expect you to have hour-long orgasms just by reading a book. You need to practice. What, after all, could be more fun than practicing something that gives you and your partner intense pleasure?

Producing orgasms is much easier than learning to play the violin, use a computer, or even play golf. How many people do you know who have given pleasure much priority in their lives, or spent much time learning to better experience and produce pleasure? After just a bit of practice, you will notice that you can either have or produce much more intense orgasms than you previously could. You might even be able to produce a "sweet sound" your first time out.

We hope that you are able to read this book with an open mind and that you take its ideas as ways to add more fun to your life. The ideas and information in this book are based on research, and we approach sensuality as scientists, yet we have had (and are having) wonderful, pleasurable experiences in this pursuit. Pleasure and research are not mutually exclusive. We do not consider ourselves therapists (not that therapists can't play an important role in people's lives), but explorers and facilitators. Therefore, there's no reason to stop doing any of the fun sexual activities you're already doing; we're not "shouldists" or moralists. This book simply gives you more options, offering proven techniques and ideas that can add more pleasure to your life.

There are a couple of other things to keep in mind as you read this book. We believe that all parties involved in sexual acts should be consenting and in agreement at all times. We also believe that it is important to deliberately plan pleasure. Many people believe that fun and pleasure should be spontaneous. Spontaneity is, of course, great when it happens, but you may have to wait a long time before it does, especially once a relationship is no longer new. In our experience, the more deliberate steps that you take to plan fun and pleasure, the more spontaneous fun and pleasure results. By practicing and deliberately training yourself and your partner to feel more via the EMO methods described in this book, you will open yourselves up to much more pleasure. Other sexual acts, such as intercourse and oral sex, will become vastly more pleasurable as well. In fact, we believe that your whole life will improve, because this work hones your communication skills, which are so important to all aspects of an effective life.

We have successfully taught this material to groups, couples, and individuals for the past twenty years. This is the first attempt that we have made to put this information into the form of a book. We are not sure how much you will be able to take from the written word, which is very different than working directly with facilitators, and we assume that some folks will get more than others from this book. But we've attempted to structure this book much like our classes. When we teach, we usually have a specific agenda, and some material is presented before other material. We're also guided by the goals of our individual students. Because we don't know your specific goals, we have attempted to put this material in the order and form that will aid the general student of sensuality. You are on your own here, and you are free to skip around to the chapters that interest you most, although we do recommend that you read the book from beginning to end. The choice is yours.

Although we just mentioned a "general" student of sensuality, this person probably does not really exist. Everyone has unique desires and goals. Our goal is for you to become an artist at doing and coming, and art is about individual creativity. It is our wish that you digest the information in this book and then take off, using your own style and creativity. In fact, we debated whether to use the words "Art" or "Science" in the book's title. We compromised, because giving and receiving EMOs is really both an art *and* a science. Once you understand and become adept at the techniques and science of doing, it will become second nature to you. At that point, your creativity will emerge, and the artist in you will develop.

## ✍ How the Book Is Structured ✍

This book has four major parts. The first, "Before Foreplay," consists of three chapters. The first presents some basic ideas, definitions, and terminology that help you understand EMOs and how to best relate to the information in the rest of the book. The second chapter explores the roles of people's cultural influences and prejudices in their sexuality, and the third chapter discusses the benefits of one person taking an active role in a sexual experience while the other takes a passive role.

The second part, "Foreplay," has three chapters that help you prepare for practicing EMO techniques. The first chapter describes some differences between men and women and helps you better understand each partner's perspective. The second chapter is about knowing your body. It provides a series of exercises that teach you to love yourself more, to feel more, and to determine how and where you prefer to be touched. The clitoris, that all-important player in orgasm, is also discussed here. The third chapter teaches you about the art of seduction and how to be a better kisser.

You will then be ready to go onto the "Play" part, which also has three chapters. The first chapter tells you about doing a woman as well as doing a man. The second chapter teaches you about the ways we've discovered that best help people communicate with their partners about sex and gives you ideas for training your partner. Finally, the last chapter offers more doing techniques, including different positions, the use of fantasy, and how to come together. The book's final section, "Coming Down," deliberately brings you down from the rest of the book with a description of heat cycles and important information on genital diseases and safe sex.

We've presented the material in this order to follow the pattern in which you should approach learning to have EMOs. You start with your partner's mind; then you seduce and do their body; and, finally, you bring them back down. Throughout this book, you will encounter examples and stories about our students, our friends, and ourselves. They're all true, but we haven't used anyone's real names (except our own), for obvious reasons. If any of these examples resemble your own story, that's because they're true, present-day human experiences.

## A Note on Language

Vera and I (Steve) usually use the plural pronoun *we* throughout this book, except for the occasional *I* when it's appropriate. Although I'm the one who's touching the keyboard and doing the typing (when Vera has no better use for my fingers), this book is a joint endeavor, and Vera has had as much input on it as I have.

Often, we've used generally accepted sexual words, such as *intercourse* and *ejaculation*. Occasionally, where we feel it works best, we've used their four-letter equivalents. We've also used the words *pussy* and *cock*, interspersed with *genitals, penis*, and *vagina*. Since these are the words that many people use in daily life, we felt we should do the same in this book. We do not wish to offend anyone, and we hope that these words will be acceptable to you.

*Before Foreplay*

# CHAPTER 1

# *What Is an EMO?*

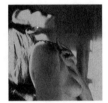

All orgasm begins in the mind, so that is where we will begin our journey. In this chapter, we will describe extended massive orgasm (EMO) and how it compares to the common conception of orgasm. We'll also delve into the underlying mental patterns that can influence orgasm. We'll describe consciousness and how we use our awareness to get or avoid our goals. Each partner's viewpoints and responsibilities also affect orgasm, so we'll spend some time on those topics as well. Finally, because sensuality, not just sexuality, plays a key role in orgasm, we'll discuss how those two concepts differ.

## ◢◢ Consciousness and Orgasm ◣◣

According to *Webster's Dictionary, consciousness* means to be "awake to our surroundings, to be aware." To be conscious is to be aware that we are awake to our
surroundings. Other animals are awake to their surroundings, but we don't
generally believe that they are conscious.

The human body receives millions of bits of information each second
through our five senses. We are only conscious of, or able to put our attention
on, a maximum of forty bits per second, and the amount is usually less.[1]
Therefore, we are only conscious of approximately one out of the millions of
sensations that we experience every second. The rest of the sensations are sub-
liminal; that is, they are below the threshold necessary to trigger a conscious
perception. Instead, they affect us subconsciously.

According to Marvin Minsky's *The Society of Mind*, there is just not
enough room or capacity in our short-term memory for us to become conscious of more information.[2] Our "hard disk" fills up quickly. If we were
conscious of all the sensations bombarding us, overload would cause us to
short-circuit.

We are usually conscious of those sensations that have gone through
some kind of change over time. According to Eric Haseltine's article
"Brainworks," published in *Discover Magazine*, "Your brain is so obsessed
with identifying changes in the environment that it ignores similarities."[3] For
example, if you go outside in the country at night, you will hear crickets making a cacophony of sound. After a short time, after you have adapted to the
noise, you will no longer hear them. The crickets have not gotten quieter. You
just don't hear them anymore because no change has occurred in the sensation. Much of thought is based on recognizing such differences. If it makes
no difference, it is not significant.

We interpret the world according to how we expect it to be. When nothing
unusual happens, our nervous system fires only a limited amount. When
something unexpected or a surprise occurs, our nerves fire rapidly. Therefore,
we are preprogrammed to select certain sensations as more important than

others even before they reach our consciousness. A sensation takes close to a half a second to become conscious.[4]

By necessity, we are able to **non-confront** (remain unconscious of) most incoming sensations. We create order in our lives with non-confrontation. We are also able to deliberately choose which sensations to confront and which to ignore. You can choose to use this ability wisely, using it to reach your goals. For example, if your goal is to learn from a teacher, you can put your attention on the teacher and become unconscious of the students next to you who are joking around. Here you are using non-confrontation in a positive way, in order to reach your goals. Yet you can also use non-confrontation unwisely, in order to avoid your goals. Two Greek gods, the brothers Thanatos and Morpheus (literally, death and sleep), represent two of the highest forms of non-confrontation. Blinking is considered a minor form of non-confrontation.

You are probably reading this book with at least fifty pounds resting on your pelvis. Before reading this last sentence, most, if not all, of you were unconscious of that fact. Our ability to be unconscious of that much weight demonstrates that our ability to be sensually unconscious is huge. Throughout most of our lives, we non-confront much that happens to us. Many people have sex without actually feeling most of the sensation available to them. They wait for the big climax at the end, while remaining unconscious of most other sensations occurring along the way, which they consider to be just foreplay and arousal.

According to our friend *Webster, orgasm* is defined as the "climax of sexual tension." But this describes the usual male ejaculatory response, in which a man tenses up his body while undergoing penile stimulation until he ejaculates. At that point, both the orgasm and the sex act are considered over. Women, whose orgasm only recently became somewhat important to society, tend to copy the orgasmic style of men.

However, the EMO that we are writing about and have demonstrated for years is much more sensational. It's about feeling your body, especially your genitals, from the very first stroke. All your attention is on perceiving pleasure. You don't compare yourself to anyone; you don't worry that you are not feeling enough or about the big climax at the end. Your orgasm starts with the first stroke and lasts as long as you are willing to experience that much pleasure. An analogy is helpful: imagine that your "normal" orgasm is the first airplane and an EMO is the space shuttle. (Note, however, that we think that any orgasm is wonderful, including the "Wright Brothers" type!) This is why when Vera saw her first demonstration of an EMO in 1976—which was the first time it was done in public—she knew right away that it was something she wanted to experience.

Orgasm begins in the mind and then manifests in the body. A person can have a wet dream without genital stimulation, but most people have been prejudiced to believe that they need to be stroked for a certain amount of time before they can have what's generally called an "orgasm." But we think that the entire universe is orgasmic. You can be orgasmic all the time; all you have to do is plug into that pleasure by putting your attention on your genitals and feeling what is happening to them. Unfortunately, people have developed many ways and reasons to avoid feeling pleasure. Many of the reasons to *not* feel pleasure are valid, given our human evolutionary past: when you're escaping a hungry lion, it's best not to be distracted by pleasure. There aren't many hungry lions out there these days, yet we still avoid feeling pleasure.

We knew a man who thought himself difficult to arouse and bring to orgasm. He met a sexy woman one day who gave him a wonderful hug. He actually ejaculated in his pants in response. This demonstrates that orgasm can begin before the first stroke. To have an orgasm requires a mental or attitude adjustment more than any physical action. As soon as your genitals feel better than any other part of your body, and as soon as your attention is on their pleasure, you are in a state of orgasm.

When we do another human being, we have to focus and put our attention on that person's orgasm. We have heard many a story about one member of a couple falling asleep while having sex. Obviously, that won't produce a great orgasm. That is an example of non-confrontation used in a negative manner, but we can also use non-confrontation in a positive manner during sex by non-confronting extraneous thoughts and sensations and keeping our attention on our partner. We also need to overcome our partner's natural tendency to non-confront sensation by paying attention to the *way* we touch. If we don't move our fingers when touching someone, or if we keep doing the same stroke over and over again, the person being touched will soon stop feeling it.

Learning to use non-confrontation in a helpful way can be scary to some of us. When we think that we will lose in a situation, avoiding that situation is a normal human response. That is why many people black out when they are in an accident. Similarly, when we undergo painful surgery, it is usually a good idea to take either a local or total anesthetic. Many people, when confronted with information about sensuality and sexuality, do not want to hear it because they fear finding out that they don't know something or are doing something wrong. They have given this area of their lives much power, which is natural: how we function in bed determines, in part, how we judge ourselves as successful human beings. Rather than taking a chance to better their lives, the risk of losing in this area makes people avoid the situation entirely. But remember that if you are reading this book, you are way ahead of the pack, and we promise that the risk you are taking is well worth your while. You are to be commended for your courage and bravery.

To help your orgasms become more intense and longer, you have to be able to approve of the orgasms you are presently experiencing. You also have to open up your mind to the possibility that your orgasms can be more intense and last longer. If you have never heard of or thought of something, that thing does not exist in your universe. Once a viewpoint or a thought has entered your mind, the possibility of its existence has entered your universe. By reading this book, the idea (and thus the possibility) of an extended massive orgasm has made its way into your mind. Communication through books, spoken words, or videos helps us to broaden our horizons. Reading about EMOs, watching a live demonstration, or viewing a video of it expands your possibilities and ability to feel more pleasure. Remember that EMOs are available to anyone with the desire and willingness to train.

Understanding this new kind of orgasm can be especially difficult for men. When it comes to pleasure, women are the first in line. Men love to be able to give pleasure to the women in their lives. But because men are so used to their old-fashioned orgasms, they have more difficulty in going for this new definition of orgasm. After all, men almost always have had some kind of an orgasm when performing coitus, while women have not. His past success is interfering with his potential pleasure—in other words, "If it's not broke, why fix it?" Yet the wonderful EMO is available to men as well.

## ✍ Viewpoints, Responsibility, ➳ and Orgasm

Now that you better understand what an EMO is and how our consciousness works, it's time to examine the ways in which we look at life and take responsibility for our life choices, both of which play significant roles in sensuality and orgasm.

Viewpoints are our thoughts. They are the tools we use to interpret our world. They are the lenses through which we see and relate to things and other people. They are rules that determine how we live our lives. As we grow older (and, hopefully, smarter), our viewpoints change and develop, but we still carry remnants of old viewpoints alongside our new ones. In this section of the book, we describe how you can develop new viewpoints while maintaining your old ones. We describe emotions and how people interpret emotions as positive or negative, depending on how much responsibility they feel they've taken for the development of these emotions. Finally, we describe the different levels of responsibility.

Everyone has viewpoints. Sometimes people's viewpoints agree, and sometimes they don't. People fight wars and destroy and kill one another over differing viewpoints. What causes this conflict is a confusion between our viewpoints and our selves. People are not their viewpoints; they merely hold viewpoints, and they choose which viewpoints they hold. An additional problem arises when viewpoints fail to keep pace with changes in our lives. This can provoke a crisis or get us into trouble. As Steven Harrison notes in his book *Doing Nothing,* crisis is the resistance to change.

How do viewpoints develop? We get our viewpoints from our parents, peers, and culture. We also acquire viewpoints through reading and the media and from our teachers and clergy. When new theories or scientific discoveries emerge, such as Einstein's theory of relativity, we may rearrange our viewpoints and thoughts. Many viewpoints develop as a result of conditioning. When we are young, we are very impressionable. For example, when our parents told us that Santa Claus brought us presents for Christmas, we probably believed them. But when we grew older and could think more rationally, we realized that our parents actually bought those presents for all those years. We still have a viewpoint about Santa Claus—it's just not the one that we were originally conditioned to have, and it's not the one that we had when we were young.

We may also hold many viewpoints at once, even if they conflict with one another. For example, you may believe that a television is a box whose pixels are stimulated by an electric current that flashes different colors on a screen. You may also believe that those pixels are real people, with real emotions and real lives playing out before you. You can hold both these viewpoints simultaneously without going crazy. These internal conflicts even express themselves in our language: "Look before you leap," we say, but we also claim, "He who hesitates is lost."

As long as your conflicting viewpoints are quite different from each other, your mind can easily handle them. Confusion occurs when differing viewpoints are too similar. I like to watch football games by turning down the sound and putting music on the stereo. I have no problem understanding what is happening in the game. However, if I watch the game with the sound off and put another football game on the radio, it becomes very confusing and difficult to understand either game.

As you read this book, you may encounter viewpoints that differ a bit from your own, and this may cause you some confusion. We don't want you to give up any of your viewpoints, but we do hope that you'll keep an open mind when you encounter an idea that conflicts with your own ideas. Both ideas could be right, depending on when and where you use them. Remember that you are not your viewpoints, and you can choose the viewpoint that best serves you in a given situation. You may have an idea of what orgasm is, but you're still free to acquire a new viewpoint on the subject.

Emotions, like viewpoints, are a human universal—everyone has them. Emotions are our conceptual responses to our sensual experiences and our previous conceptual responses. Emotions are also value judgments that we make about our experiences and responses, so we have both positive and negative emotions. We are built to experience both kinds, and a full life includes both kinds. A person who experiences primarily negative emotions is sad and depressed, but a person who *never* experiences negative emotions is dull and is also unable to feel the extremes of their positive experiences. Such a person could not fully experience the sad beauty of Shakespeare's tragedies or the delicious fear of a good horror movie. Humans want to experience as much as they can, and this means appreciating both positive and negative emotions. The best way to handle a negative emotion is to realize that it is the proper response to what you have experienced. Realize that you are a human being who can feel both pleasure and sadness. Do not fight your negative feelings, for the more attention and energy you use to resist them, the more power they have over you.

We perceive an experience as positive or negative according to how much responsibility we believe we've had for creating that experience. Parachuting out of a small airplane might be terrifying if the plane has lost its engines, but it might be delightful if you've deliberately chosen to go skydiving. In fact, many people have described skydiving to us as one of the most wonderful things they have ever done. Some have even said that it was better than an orgasm. They probably never experienced a full EMO, but you get the point. The only difference between the experiences is that in the first you felt victimized and felt no responsibility, and in the second you felt responsible for creating the experience.

The highest level of human awareness, which can be called enlightenment, nirvana, or oneness with the universe, is the one at which you take total responsibility for everything. You realize you are the divine or "great spirit." You are one with the universe, and so is everybody and everything else. The lowest level of human awareness is the one at which you refuse to take responsibility for anything. Everything happens to you by luck or chance. You are a total victim. There are many levels between these extremes, of course. You can choose to relate to your experiences from any level of responsibility, and because people can hold more than one viewpoint on a given subject, you don't have to stay at any specific level. Sometimes it's fun to be a victim—for example, when you're a victim of pleasure. At other times, you can enjoy being more responsible by deliberately creating new ideas and experiences.

A person's responses to you depend upon the level of responsibility and awareness that you communicate from, as well as their own level of responsibility and awareness. If the two of you are on or near the same level, you'll relate just fine. If you are one level above them, you can help them see new possibilities. They may respond with a "Wow!" Being one level above someone is a fine position for teaching. However, when you're communicating with or trying to teach someone who is two levels below you, you may encounter problems. They may hear what you say but be unable to understand it or why you said it. They may respond with "What?" If you're three or more levels above someone you're trying to teach or communicate with, they'll get angry with you. They may believe that they're victims, feel that they're not responsible for the mess that they think they're in, or blame the government, their lousy childhood, or any other handy villain. When you tell them that they *are* responsible for their situation, they may eventually benefit from that information, but their first reaction will be hostility toward you. It's dangerous to teach from a distance of more than three levels, as some people may actually react violently—that is what happened to Jesus Christ, Gandhi, and Martin Luther King, Jr.

In general, taking responsibility for your experiences allows you to perceive them more pleasurably. It also enables you to feel more control over your life. Responsibility enables you to change your life and steer it in the direction that you choose. If you live as a victim by choosing not to take responsibility, you will have great difficulty in steering your life in the direction that you want.

The essence of the victim's viewpoint is disagreement with the way that life is. If you want control of your life, you must be in agreement with the way that your life is, or you must make your life agree with you (which is usually harder). By choosing responsibility, you're choosing control. A great analogy is that of driving a car on an icy road. The car goes into a skid. In order to regain control of the car, you have to turn the steering wheel into the skid. If you fight the skid by turning the wheel in the opposite direction, you only make things worse. By being in agreement with the skid, you are able to regain control of the vehicle. By being in agreement with your life, you have chosen responsibility and are able to take your life in any direction you choose.

## ✍ Sensuality out of Sexuality ✍

To help you better understand EMOs, we would like to explain the difference between sensuality and sexuality. Sensuality is about giving pleasure to the body or mind through the senses. The key word here is _pleasure_. Sensuality includes all five of our senses: hearing, seeing, smelling, tasting, and touching. It also includes the sixth sense, which is any use of conceptual thought to enhance pleasure. Because this book is about orgasm, we're most concerned with the sense of touch. Sexuality, meanwhile, is the physiological function that pertains to reproduction brought about by insemination of the female by the male through penile penetration of the vagina.

Lynn Margulis's and Dorion Sagan's book _What Is Sex?_ explains that there are three original types of sex, which evolved among bacteria. The earliest sex was **transgenic sex**, which evolved in bacteria or prokaryotes. It involves the movement of genes from a donor source (bacterium, virus, chemical solution, etc.) to a live recipient bacterium. This genetic movement, present at the dawn of life, provided an important means of survival for all subsequent life. (Today's biotechnology revolution exploits this tendency of bacteria to donate and receive each other's genes, regardless of species.) The second type of sex to evolve was **hypersex**. All familiar life forms, including animals, plants, and fungi, come from hypersex. It is the permanent merging, through symbiosis, to produce organisms with genes from more than one source. One bacterium enters another and grows and reproduces inside forever. Permanent unions among originally separate bacteria led to new life forms. All our cells resulted from this original bacterial union or hypersex. The third type of sex, **meiotic sex**, evolved in organisms that had previously evolved by bacterial hypersex. Meiotic sex produces the animal sperm and eggs, or the plant or fungal spores, by meiosis. In meiosis, the number of chromosomes is halved; fertilization follows and restores the full number of chromosomes. This process, and its accompanying genital-to-genital friction, is what people commonly think of as sex.

All three types of sex share a common element: they involve some form of DNA exchange. (So Bill Clinton didn't lie, at least in a technical sense, when he claimed he "did not have sex with that woman.") Sexuality is a goal-oriented activity. The goal is reproduction, and the occurrence of pleasure is only incidental. Sensuality, however, is not goal oriented. If there is a goal, it is to feel wonderful sensation at every moment of the experience. Pleasure is of the utmost importance.

Sexuality is, obviously, part of our lives, and everyone alive today, excluding those born through artificial insemination, is the result of a successful sexual act. However, the ability to give and receive exceptional sensual pleasure must be learned. We are all able to eat, after all, but that doesn't make us gourmet cooks. There is a big difference between creating and enjoying wonderfully prepared dishes, and just stuffing our faces with whatever's at hand. Hunger and digestion are, like sex, natural physiological processes, but their only goal is to replenish our bodies with nutrients and calories. If we wish to take the utmost pleasure from eating and digesting, we have to learn the art of cooking and preparing food that titillates our taste buds.

When considering the differences between sexuality and sensuality, another useful analogy is music. Our sense of hearing is a basic physiological function, and music developed because we have the natural ability to hear sound. To sensually appreciate an entire piece of music, you must listen to all its sounds and notes, from the beginning to the end. You can't just listen to a few notes or wait to hear the end of the piece. Yet, when most people have sex, they just go through the motions to reach the last few strokes, when they experience a brief orgasmic "sneeze." No one goes to the opera or symphony to listen to just the last eight notes. In order for you to enjoy the end of a composition, or a sexual act, you must listen to all its notes. The accumulated pleasure that you have enjoyed throughout your listening experience makes the ending much more enjoyable.

Even the word *foreplay* implies that activity before intercourse is just work that has to be done in order to reach the really fun "play" part of sex. In reality, the whole experience can be the fun part, and that is the goal of the true sensualist. In the rest of this book, we've used *sexuality* and *sensuality* interchangeably, because we don't think that sexuality means only intercourse. Instead, it describes a complete sensual experience.

Consciousness, responsibility, and the difference between sexuality and sensuality are topics that we always discuss at the start of our EMO courses. We do this because it gives students a basic understanding of our viewpoint and provides them with concepts that will help them understand how EMO exercises and techniques work. Hopefully, your appetite has now been whetted a bit, and you're ready to dive into the rest of the book.

# CHAPTER 2

# Prejudice and Pain

## How Our Ideas Affect Our Orgasms

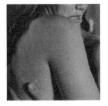

*I*n this chapter, we meet the main players in any EMO—
you and your partner. As we noted in the previous chapter, our previous experiences and viewpoints play a
significant role in determining how we live our sensual lives,
so here we discuss the role of prejudice and how it interferes
with EMOs. We also examine society's influence on our
sensual lives, explaining why pain is perceived as positive
and why so many people find it difficult to pursue pleasure.

## ✍ Prejudice ✍

We judge our viewpoints as either "good" or "bad" based upon how they affect our goals. If our viewpoint prevents us from reaching our goals, we can say that it's a bad viewpoint, at least in this particular circumstance. If the viewpoint helps us reach our goals, we can say that it's a good viewpoint, at least for this situation. Viewpoints that don't affect our goals at all aren't good or bad; they're neutral.

A prejudice is a bad viewpoint and prevents us from reaching our goals. In this section, we explore prejudice, especially commonly held sexual prejudices that interfere with achieving a better sex life, and explain how they affect us.

Prejudices tend to limit sensual experiences. As soon as we were born, we knew what we liked and didn't like. We preferred to be dry and warm and surrounded by pleasant odors; we didn't like being wet, cold, and smelly. So from the get-go, we had judgments about sensual experiences that determined their value to us. Prejudice is different than these judgments, which were based upon information that we received from the world around us. Prejudice is a pre-judgment based upon a scarcity of information.

Greed and stinginess are prejudices caused by scarcity of money, but belief in the abundance of money causes generosity. Meanness is caused by scarcity of kindness, but belief in the abundance of kindness causes us to behave kindly. When a person chooses scarcity over abundance, or chooses to believe in scarcity rather than abundance, he is sure to lead a poor, limited life. Sometimes our prejudices agree with later judgments that we form once we have sufficient information; these prejudices generally prove themselves benign. Often, however, prejudices actually *cause* judgments, and thus lead us to make bad decisions that limit our lives.

Here's a story that illustrates how prejudices develop from lack of information. In the 1960s, Joe Pyne, an ex-Marine with a wooden leg who ran a Jerry Springer-type talk show, interviewed Frank Zappa, the longhaired musician who led the group The Mothers of Invention. Pyne said to Zappa, "You have long hair. You must be a woman." Zappa responded, "You have a wooden leg. You must be a table." This story might seem funny or silly, but it really shows how foolish prejudices are.

People have prejudices about all facets of their lives, and almost everyone has some prejudices, whether they're about race, gender, food, size, appearance, or another subject. Most people also have prejudices about sex. Some people think, for example, that it's more important for men to have orgasms than women. Some people also believe that only men need to be excited and physically engorged before intercourse. And some people believe that there's only one kind of orgasm, the tensed-up, "squirt, squirt, squirt" variety described by Kinsey.

These prejudices are, like Joe Pyne's, based on a lack of information. Here are the facts. A woman who has coitus who hasn't been stimulated and engorged before penetration doesn't experience as much pleasure as a woman who has been properly engorged. Very likely, she experiences discomfort, and perhaps even pain. Since the human race began, men have inserted their penises into women without knowing that women need to be engorged to take the most pleasure from the act. (We don't want to blame men here; we're only discussing how prejudiced most people are about male and female engorgement.) If a woman is engorged, there's less likelihood of pain and injury, and there's also a greater chance that her clitoris can engage in the in-out movement of intercourse, because engorgement tends to move the clitoris toward her introitus (vaginal opening). Of course, many women do enjoy intercourse, but many more would enjoy it if they were properly stimulated and engorged first.

Let's examine another of these prejudices, the idea that men's orgasms are the most important. It's hard to believe that people hold this viewpoint, given that it's so sexist. But the lack of information on female orgasm explains why the prejudice persists. Many women either don't experience orgasm at all or don't have orgasms each time they have sex. Men, on the other hand, generally have orgasms with every sex act. Prostitution, considered the "world's oldest profession," is based upon causing male orgasms. Only in the last part of the twentieth century did female orgasm become a topic of research and open discussion. For reproductive purposes alone, male orgasm may indeed be more important, but even that point is debatable, because men who leak seminal fluid before ejaculation and then pull out have, more than once, caused pregnancy.

What about the third prejudice that we've mentioned, the idea that there's only one kind of orgasm? As we've previously mentioned, orgasm is actually a state that begins in the mind, just as it does in a wet dream. An orgasm can last for a few seconds or hours. Relaxing instead of tensing helps people to feel more, not less, and they feel it for a longer time. These longer, intense orgasms are quite different from the usual "crotch sneeze" that most people experience. If you're prejudiced about orgasm, if you believe that it arrives only after a period of tension and is limited only to the climax of that tension, your mind is closed to the idea of extended orgasms, which can be far more intense than anything you've felt before.

Choosing an abundant amount of information helps you make better decisions. Prejudices, created by choosing stingy amounts of information, limit your life in all of the areas that they affect. It's good to know your own prejudices. Only then will you have any hope of opening your mind and life to more experiences and opportunities. Knowing your prejudices also benefits your survival and your happiness. If you're prejudiced against women and don't realize it, you might encounter deep trouble in your relationships, if indeed relationships are even possible for you.

Prejudice against women informs many sexual prejudices. In American society and most other cultures, prejudice has made women into second-class citizens. Such prejudice is caused by a lack of information. As the women's movement and technological advancements in communication move across the world, women may begin to shake free of such prejudice, assuming leadership roles and leading men and themselves into more pleasurable lives. Such changes have sexual ramifications as well; women's engorgement, hopefully, will be considered as important as men's, and their full-body, extended, intense orgasms will come to define "orgasm" for all sensual people.

## ☞ Pain on a Pedestal ☜

In the previous chapter, we described how we obtain our viewpoints from our parents, peers, teachers, and culture. American society is an agglomeration of many different cultures, of course, but one of the most prominent threads in our country's heritage is Puritanism. The "Puritan work ethic," which directly or indirectly influences everyone who lives in our culture, creates a prevailing belief that suffering and pain are noble and pleasure is sinful and harmful.

The Puritan work ethic teaches that we must pay in advance for any pleasure that we get. Puritanism also teaches that we were born in sin and thus must pay for pleasure with pain. In order to get the evening off, we have to pay by working at least eight hours during the day and driving twice through rush-hour traffic. To get the weekend off, we have to work the rest of the week. To get two weeks off in summer, we must, along with everyone else and his uncle, work fifty straight weeks. We must work until we are senior citizens, and only then can we retire to do what we supposedly wanted to do all along.

This "pay first, pleasure later" mentality is one that has brainwashed us all. You can notice it in all areas of life, if you pay attention. It's apparent in religion. For example, of all the images we have of Jesus Christ, the most visible one is that of Christ nailed to the cross, bleeding and dying in anguish. Whether you believe in Jesus Christ or not, many wonderful, joyous stories were written about him and his deeds, yet the most ubiquitous image of him depicts his painful death. We live in a society that puts pain on a pedestal and even worships it.

Pain is also considered more important than pleasure in work. It's okay to take off the day if you're suffering. You can call and say that you've broken your leg or can hardly breathe due to flu, and everyone is okay with that. But what would happen if you called and said that you couldn't work today because you were having so much fun with your lover that the two of you wanted to stay in bed all day? Your employer would probably tell you not to bother coming in ever again.

Pain is emphasized by the media as well. Although there are some sensual shows on television, most of them are on expensive cable stations late at night.

Far more shows feature violence and pain than sensuality. Most cartoons that our children grow up watching show many violent scenes every minute. Characters are squashed like pancakes, run over, blown up, drowned, and mutilated in all kinds of inventive ways. News shows focus on people who experienced the most pain that day and detail how, where, and why that pain occurred.

Society also conditions us to think that sex is bad for us. When we do have it, society teaches, we should do it in the dark and not talk about it. Masturbation is considered sinful by some religions; in the past, people were taught that it made hair grow on their palms, caused pimples, and made them go blind. Even today, many of our students who masturbate still feel they shouldn't. They think that there must be something wrong with them if they masturbate, and they feel guilty. Guilt arises when we do something according to one of our rules or viewpoints but then later judge ourselves according to another viewpoint that we hold. Margo Woods, writing in *Tantra and Self Love,* says that the word *masturbation* comes from the Latin *man*(u)*sturprare*. *Manu* means "hand," and *stuprum* means "dishonor, defilement, a disgrace." *Turbare* is also part of this word; in relation to *stuprum,* it means "to disturb, confuse." It's related to the words *stupid* and *stupefaction.* No wonder that masturbation is such a negatively charged topic for us. This book is about pleasure—we don't want to focus too much on guilt. However, it's necessary to recognize that the baggage some of us carry around causes us to resist pleasure.

A simple experiment demonstrates that most people give priority to pain over pleasure. If you want to strike up a lively conversation at a party, you can bring up your knee operation or triple bypass surgery, and more than likely people will jump in and enthusiastically describe their own pains. If, however, you bring up your last wonderful orgasm, most people will look at you funny and walk away as soon as they can.

All of us were conceived by at least one orgasm (you know your father had one, but whether your mother did is questionable). We were conceived by the act of pleasure, yet somehow the pain lobby has trumped this ecstasy. Sex before marriage is considered sinful by most religions. Sex after marriage should be, in some religious teachings, limited to reproductive purposes only.

Stories of childbirth emphasize pain, not joy, although we've met many women who reported feeling orgasmic while giving birth. Is it any wonder that pleasure and sensuality are so difficult to achieve?

Society also teaches us that pain and pleasure are opposites. Pain is supposed to repel, and pleasure is supposed to attract. Yet pain and pleasure share one quality: they command all of your attention. When you're in pain, you can think of nothing else. Sometimes the only way to stop noticing the pain you feel is to start feeling a new, stronger pain somewhere else—if you want to stop feeling your bad back, smash your thumb with a hammer. When you experience great pleasure, as in orgasm, you are totally absorbed, and you forget all your troubles and problems. It's difficult to go for pleasure when you hurt and feel awful. But if you can, the pain miraculously disappears, at least during the course of your pleasure. Pain and pleasure both have the ability to distract you from whatever else is happening in your life.

There's one benefit of living in a pain-oriented society, as opposed to a pleasure-oriented one where nudity and sensuality are open: We can experience more eroticism. Eroticism results from breaking taboos or minor social rules. Living in our society, with all of its regulations, means living among an abundance of rules and taboos that can be violated. This is why it's more erotic to put your hand on your girlfriend's knee under the tablecloth in a fancy restaurant than to do the same thing at home in front of the television. If sex and pleasure were open topics, there would be fewer rules to break and, as a result, less eroticism.

We have seen why so many people in our society are afraid to go for more pleasure in their lives. Given the lack of information about sex and the rules against talking and communicating about pleasure, it is no wonder that we have so many prejudices and difficulties in exploring our sensuality.

☙

# CHAPTER 3

# Cause and Effect

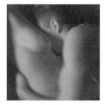

**M**any people hold a common prejudice: They believe that pleasure should be spontaneous and that they should not talk about pleasure that they plan to have. We, on the other hand, believe that planning for pleasure is perfectly valid and, in fact, adds joy to your life.

One of the best ways to deliberately plan pleasure is to choose an active or passive role in a sensual act. We call the active and passive roles "cause" and "effect." These roles help you create the highest possible level of pleasure and orgasm.

When you and your partner assume these roles, both of you focus all your attention on one person's orgasm. We call this "doing." Doing is the manual stimulation of a person's genitals, and it also refers to the seduction and romancing of their mind before any physical contact occurs. Doing shouldn't be confused with intercourse.

In order to help you better understand doing, this chapter defines cause and effect. We explain that effect always precedes cause, even though most people think that cause must come first. We show you how you can assume the role of cause or effect and explain the difficulties and pleasures involved in each role. Finally, we describe how the two roles are created in the same way.

According to *Webster's*, *effect* means "the result of an action by some agent and cause that is that agent's action." They really refer to imaginary links that connect the differences we sense.[5] In other words, there is no absolute connection between cause and effect, only a statistical connection. As we noted in the previous chapter's "Consciousness" section, our senses work by noticing differences. If differences don't occur, we don't sense anything. For example, if we are in a room with a woman wearing strong perfume, we notice the smell at first. After we are in the room a while, we don't smell the perfume anymore. That's because our olfactory system no longer perceives any change. We've become "used to" the smell.

This example also serves to illustrate the ways that we search for cause based upon effect. We notice the smell of perfume (the effect) first. Probably we conclude that the perfume smell comes from the woman in the room (the cause), but we can't be certain about the cause—it might have been another woman, or maybe someone spilled a perfume bottle. We perceive effect first, then we create a cause that fits that effect. We assume that cause precedes effect, so we create causes that we think are responsible for the effects that we notice. There may not be any clear connections between an effect and a cause, but based upon our life experience, we automatically try to create causes. We do certain things in order to feel a certain way. Sometimes we might be better served if we decided to feel the way we hoped to feel, and then did what we really wanted to do. For example, instead of needing money or a relationship to feel happy, we should decide to feel happy first. In this way, we aren't so dependent on outside influences or causes to reach a desired emotional state. It is a holistic rather than a linear view of life.

We assign names to each of the EMO partners according to the roles they play in the encounter. The "doer," the active participant, is the one who "takes cause" or "is cause." The "doee," the passive participant, is the one who "is effect." Basically, these names are assigned based on who takes responsibility in the sensual encounter. The one who is cause takes responsibility for the experience; the one who is effect does not.

Here's an example. Suppose you take a tour of London. Your tour guide is cause. The guide takes you to places that they know, and you feel cared for. You, meanwhile, are effect. When you become a "doing" artist, you are like this guide. You tell the person whom you do that they only need to be effect. All your partner has to do is feel pleasure and communicate that pleasure in an enjoyable way. Both you and your partner, in your roles of cause and effect, focus your attention upon the orgasm. This allows the orgasm to reach its maximum potential.

Of course, this is easier said than done in our society, where "being done" may have fearful connotations. People are afraid of being total effect because it puts them in a vulnerable position. You can see this even in our language: It's much better to "fuck" someone than to "get fucked" or "be fucked over." Effect is a place where someone can take advantage of you and do harmful things to you. If you are at effect, you must be able to trust that the person at cause will not do you any harm because you are surrendering your body into their hands.

People may be less afraid of taking the cause position, but it also has a negative side. People may be eager to be cause at first, but after a while, they can start to feel used. They may think and say things such as, "Why do I always have to be the responsible one? Why can't someone do it to *me* for a change?" I lived in Italy for a while and had a VW van. Friends from America often visited me, and I was glad to be able to drive them around and show them the sights. Once, when I was driving and my passengers were laughing and having fun, I became upset that I always had to be the chauffeur, even though I'd eagerly agreed to play tour guide. This is a classic example of choosing to be cause and then feeling used. Partway through the experience, you might decide that you no longer want to be cause and want to be put at effect.

As we've mentioned earlier, when most people talk about sex, they're referring to sexual intercourse. (Just ask Bill Clinton.) Neither party claims to be cause or effect; indeed, no one talks very much at all. He wonders what she feels, worries about whether he should pay more attention to her pleasure, and fears that if he does he'll come too soon. Meanwhile, she wonders why she doesn't feel more, wonders if he's being pleasured, and wonders if she should fake an orgasm. The goal of this kind of intercourse is simultaneous orgasm. You have better odds trying to shoot flying ducks at night with straw in a windstorm. It's not going to happen, and there are much better ways to orgasm.

Why do cause and effect ensure the best orgasms? If one partner is at effect, they are in a vulnerable position where harm could befall them, but they're also in the position where the most pleasure is available to them. Just as it's difficult to really twist your own arm, it's difficult to give yourself overwhelming pleasure. This is because you always know your own motivations, and since you know what you're up to, you can't seduce and tease yourself as effectively as someone who knows how to seduce you and wants to please you. To experience intense pleasure, you have to put yourself into someone else's hands and be a "pleasure victim." Simultaneous orgasm, in an EMO encounter, happens every time both partners put their attention on one partner at a time. Both partners experience that orgasm together, one as cause, the other as effect, and that is a true "simultaneous" orgasm. (If you wish to learn more about simultaneous orgasm, read the "Coming Together" section in Chapter 9.)

You must, of course, be a superb "cause person" to convince a person to put himself or herself into the vulnerable effect state. This means you must make your partner feel safe and assured and let them know that you are confident and they are in good hands. If you are a good doer, your ultimate goal is to seduce the "doee" to surrender their central nervous system into your hands.

Good "effect people" know how to play the cause role as well as their own. If you are unable or unwilling to be cause, to put your total attention onto another person's body and pleasure, you'll find it difficult to surrender your own body into your partner's hands. You'll believe that your partner feels as you do, and because you know you can't trust yourself, you won't trust them, either. But to the extent that you can be cause, you can be effect. If you want to have great EMOs, you'll benefit from putting your partner at total effect rather than always being at total effect yourself.

We knew a woman who trained to have EMOs but who only had "good" orgasms that weren't as intense as she had hoped. She also felt bored when she did her husband. We told her how she could have more fun doing him; those ideas worked for her, and, as a result, she was able to give him more pleasure. At the same time, her orgasmic ability expanded and she felt more pleasure than she ever believed she could. She had learned to be better effect by being better cause.

When you are at cause, you must create the space for seduction, create the objects in that space, and create the time to share pleasure in that space. For example, let's consider a couple on a date. He wants to take her to dinner, so he chooses a restaurant. He "creates" the space, as well as the objects in it: the fine food, waiters, tables, silverware, etc. He creates the time, too: say, 7:30 on a Friday night. The woman, who is in the role of effect, also needs to create the space, the objects in it, and the time to enjoy them, but then she needs to forget she's done all that. She may have told her boyfriend that she wants to have dinner on Friday night at her favorite restaurant. When he takes her out, however, she forgets that she's said this so that she can step into the role of effect and simply enjoy the experience.

Here's another example. Suppose you are cooking for a dinner party. You are at cause. Many people who have cooked all day don't want to eat when dinnertime arrives. All the guests, however, who are at effect, enjoy the food. You may put your own portion in a bag and freeze it. The next week, you come home late from work. You're hungry, so you put the frozen meal in the microwave. A few minutes later, you have a gourmet meal to enjoy, and you feel at effect.

Later, in the "Training and Communication" chapter, we describe how you can train your partner from either the cause or the effect position. Once you become familiar with how to do and how to get done, you will find that taking either the cause or the effect positions can be very gratifying. In the next chapter, we will tell you about some obstacles that can hinder both men and women as they learn more about the roles of cause and effect. We will show you how to best handle these obstacles, and we'll tell you more about the philosophies underlying EMO techniques.

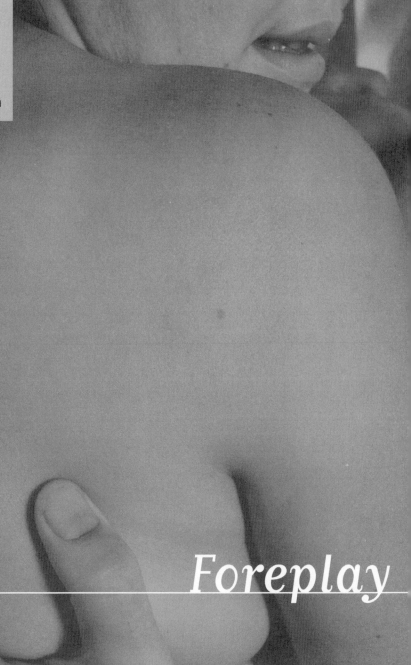

# part two

*Foreplay*

# CHAPTER 4

# Know Yourself
# and Your Partner

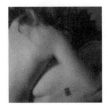

*I* (Steve) got married for the first time when I was twenty-one, to my college sweetheart. I was madly in love, but I did not know the first thing about pleasing a woman. We were both virgins when we met. We spent the first two years of marriage in Italy, where I was in medical school. Being in a foreign country enabled us to stick together and enjoy each other. However, when we came back to the United States, we grew farther and farther apart. She became progressively angrier with me, and I did not know what to do to make her happy. We divorced after four years of marriage.

When I met Vera, I was older and wiser. I knew the importance of pleasuring a woman and some techniques to accomplish that. Vera was more than thirteen years older than I, and neither of us matched the image of a prospective spouse, but we were still sexually attracted to each other despite the fact that Vera was married and I was in love with another woman at that time. We did sensual research together, but considered each other to be friends as opposed to lovers. We later became lovers and still continued being friends, and Vera's pleasure was always considered top priority in our relationship. This has not changed in the twenty years that we have known each other, except that we have continually learned to become better at it. We have not met many, if any, couples who have the passion and romance that we have. I have learned the importance of pleasure, and she has learned to place her happiness before any anger or desire for revenge on men. We both feel that our communication and the fact that we talk about everything that happens have made our relationship a success.

To have a successful relationship and to have and give EMOs, it's essential to know the fears, hopes, and desires of both players in the encounter: yourself and your partner. So we offer you a short description of most people's basic fears about sexuality, along with practical suggestions for dealing with those fears. We also describe some differences between men and women. Some viewpoints presented here may be new to you (and hopefully they won't offend you!). If you can understand some of the basic similarities and differences between yourself and your partner, you'll be better able to seduce and please your partner. For many women, anger is a problem in learning to have EMOs. For many men, feeling used or tired of being the "cause" can be a problem in learning to give EMOs. We discuss these problems and show how EMOs can actually benefit both men and women once they've learned to "win" with each other rather than lose. The best relationships are those in which the woman feels gratified and loved. Creating such relationships is a dance between men and women, and this chapter shows you some of the basic steps in that dance.

## ◟◞ **Fear and Approval** ◟◞

Most people have some fears and apprehensions about sex and their sexual performance. That's perfectly natural, given that our society doesn't promote sensuality as a noble virtue. Society also manipulates sensuality, presenting images of beautiful models in product advertisements who make us feel inadequate. Most people don't talk about sex even when they're doing it, and many people do it in the dark. Little information about sex is available unless you research the topic for yourself; as a result, most people are ignorant about sex and only know what their (equally ignorant) friends and the media have told them about it.

Since you've bought this book, we assume that you're eager to expand your horizons, overcome obstacles, and push past such social prejudices. The first step in doing this is realizing that the only proper yardstick to measure yourself and your sexual performance *is* yourself. You are a perfect you, despite what the media says. Your fears and worries are normal, but you can overcome them by paying attention to your experiences and remaining focused on what happens to you. Attention and focus are the essence of sensuality, because they enable you to feel more pleasure. Each time you become fearful, remind yourself to return to the present moment and feel the sensation at hand. Fear is an emotion concerned with the future. As long as you remain concerned with the present, fear can't sweep you away. We tell students to put their fear and excitement into their genitals.

By reading this book, you've already taken a huge step toward bettering your life and learning to have pleasurable experiences. Your desire for knowledge will cancel out many of your fears. Remember that the only person who can feel what you feel *is* you. You can decide to approve of who you are and what you're doing, and you can also decide to approve of the sensations that you're now experiencing. Approval is the only way that those sensations will start to feel better and become more intense.

If you're currently experiencing a lot of fear, you might flip to the next chapter in which we provide specific sensual exercises that help you to focus on your body, approve of your body, and love yourself more. The "Training and Communication" chapter is also helpful, because it suggests wonderful ways to talk to your partner before, during, and after sex.

## Anger or Happiness?
### EMO's Benefits for Women

Why do people get angry? Among both women and men, anger results when we believe that a personal right has been violated. Everyone believes that they have rights, all kinds of rights, whether it is the right to breathe or, in some countries, the right to vote. We usually don't think about these rights as long as they are not threatened, but when someone violates a right, we notice it immediately and get angry. This is a formula for anger. For example, when someone cuts you off in traffic, your right to a smooth journey has been violated and you usually get angry.

It is almost universal that women are angry with men. Although they are numerically in the majority, women have been treated like a second-class minority for thousands of years, ever since agricultural societies first developed.[6] One fact that is common among all oppressed minorities is that they are pissed off, angry with those whom they consider their oppressors. Some women are angrier at men than other women are, but because of human history, anger is inevitable. Women usually take this anger out on the men closest to them. (To some extent, her anger is a compliment. It means she's close to you. If she were angry with someone else, you might be jealous.) Men, of course, also get angry. They notice when their rights are violated, just as women do. But men have not been told to consider themselves second-class citizens, so their anger toward women isn't so inflamed (except in psychologically disturbed men).

If a woman doesn't get what she wants, she is unhappy. If a man does not treat her as she wants, very often she gets angry. This is also true for men, but the dynamics are somewhat different for them (and this book's primary focus is, after all, on how to please a woman). Often men are so unaware that they don't even notice when they have stepped on a woman's feet. Overcoming this lack of awareness and learning to handle anger is crucial to learning to have and produce EMOs. If a woman is angry with her partner, there is no way that she will surrender her nervous system into his hands. Anger is the enemy of turn-on and, therefore, of orgasm. Anger means that a person's attention is on their anger, not on their orgasm.

Her anger, frustration, or unhappiness can result from a misnaming of goals. Misnaming means that a person is out of agreement with the reality of their life. In essence, they are "losing." Losing happens when we are out of agreement with our current circumstances and believe that those circumstances will always be as they are right now. To win in any situation, we must be in agreement with our lives and their circumstances, so that we can feel in control of our lives and, if possible, change those circumstances. This helps us to attain our goals, and thus we win.

To win, we have two choices. We can do whatever it takes to make sure that we get what we think we want. But this can be difficult, and it involves a lot of time and effort. There's a second way to win, however: by getting into agreement with the way that our lives are right now. We can find our lives perfect, or "right," just as they are. We can realize that we may not have everything that we think we want but that our lives are great anyway. We can realize, too, that it is okay to want things; if our desire is true, we'll eventually get what we want. Being in agreement brings us happiness. With our newfound happiness, it becomes easier to attract people and experience pleasure.

Becoming happy and less angry also requires taking responsibility for our own situations. A woman, if she feels angry with a man, can overcome her anger by taking responsibility for her situation and teaching him how to treat her and gratify her. Attention is more important than gifts in this regard. A man can give a woman lots of gifts, but if his attention isn't on her when she wants it, she remains ungratified and unhappy. Most men really don't know what women want, so it is best if women take responsibility for their situations and teach the men in their lives what they *do* want.

In his book *Vital Energy*, David Simon writes that responsibility means exercising your ability to have creative responses to your emotional triggers.[7]

In terms of women's anger toward men, responsibility means that women need to have creative responses to that anger. To feel happier, a woman needs to realize that her anger is not in her best interest. It is, however, in her best interest to realize that most men are socially dumb and have to be taught to treat her in the way that she wants. She needs to decide which is more important to her: happiness or anger.

This is, of course, a difficult attitude adjustment for anyone who's in the midst of feeling miserable and angry. A woman can begin this adjustment by letting a man know immediately and in a friendly fashion when he's done something that upset her. She can realize in advance that men are often unwittingly clumsy and hurt her, and decide to do her best to inform the men whom she cares for when they act or say things that offend her. By expressing herself, she feels less temptation to get angry at him or at herself. She prevents angry thoughts from accumulating. If allowed to fester in silence, anger tends to grow.

Most women are more intuitive than most men. Women often think that men should know exactly what they want and how to treat them, without being told. This is a formula for trouble. When a man doesn't give her what she wants, she thinks that he is being mean and inattentive. In truth, he may well be inattentive, but he may also be misinformed. He probably would love to know what she wants, so that he could give it to her. If she wants attention, he probably wants to give it to her, so that he can "win" with her.

Usually men aren't trying to be mean when they don't give women what they want; they simply don't know what women want. One woman we know is married to a man who adores her. They used to go to a friend's house for dinner parties. The wife loved the way that their friend served dinner, making sure everyone had food on their plates. She decided to try her friend's style at her own dinner parties. Once, while she was occupied with their baby, she assumed that her husband would serve their guests in the same manner. He didn't. Her plate remained empty, although everyone else, including her husband, had begun eating. She was infuriated. Later, she realized that she had never told him about her new way of serving. She calmed down and told him why she was angry. Her plate has never been empty since.

A woman can also use positive reinforcement when a man does something that pleases her. Positive reinforcement is the best method for teaching or training anyone. (See the "Training from Effect" section of Chapter 8 for some ideas on how to use positive reinforcement.) She can begin to learn positive reinforcement by focusing her attention on one thing in her life that she finds positive. Once she is able to do this, she can find other positive things to focus upon and is on her way to feeling better.

Anger can also be overcome by learning to appreciate what her partner produces for her. If she can learn to appreciate whatever her partner—or anyone else, for that matter—produces for her, and feel enthusiasm and enjoyment for their gifts, more and better things and feelings will come her way in the future. (This dynamic is true for men as well as women.) An important part of women's sensual and emotional appetites is their ability to consume. To consume something well is to appreciate it to its fullest value. Of course, appreciation has to be genuine.

Hans Christian Andersen wrote a cute story called "What Father Does Is Always Right." A farmer trades a horse for a cow, the cow for a sheep, the sheep for a goose, the goose for a hen, and the hen for a bag of rotten apples. He winds up in a tavern where there are two rich gentlemen. They bet him 100 gold pieces that his wife will be pissed when he tells her what he traded the horse for. They all go to his wife together, and she meets her husband with a kiss. He relates the whole story of his trading, and she's thrilled as he tells her about each exchange because she thinks that he made the exchanges to make her happy. She is most thrilled with the bag of rotten apples, and the gentlemen have to pay the farmer 100 gold coins.

The farmer's wife was thrilled with everything that her husband produced for her, and this empowered both of them. She had no particular expectations for what he would produce. If a person has expectations but events don't turn out as expected, that person usually "loses." It's fine to have goals, and even to do what it takes to reach those goals, but if you're married to a particular outcome or set of expectations, you're setting yourself up for unhappiness. The wife in this story appreciated what her husband had done, what she had attracted for herself from him. If a person, man or woman, doesn't appreciate what they've attracted, there's little hope that more and better things will follow.

To get what you want, you must manifest your desires. But sometimes a woman does not manifest her desires, often because doubts about her attractiveness or deservingness prevent her from doing so. Her doubt cancels her desire. As a result, men (and other people) in her life who want to help her reach her desires are confused and don't know how to help. A woman who isn't manifesting her true desires and having them fulfilled may fill up on other things instead, such as material goods like food, clothing, jewelry, or even children. Women who *are* genuinely gratified often want these things too, of course, but they are a lot happier with them (and patient while waiting for them) than their turned-off sisters are. Their happiness and attractiveness attract the fulfillment of their desires.

Attraction or being attractive consists of appetite or desire, the ability to consume, and acknowledging and appreciating what was consumed. A gratified person is extremely beautiful and radiant. By acknowledging and appreciating, both men and women are able to swallow what they have consumed. This, in turn, opens them up to more goodies and makes them even more attractive.

We knew a man who was beginning a relationship with a woman he considered very beautiful. She wanted him to take her to the opera. She wanted him to take her in a limousine, and she wanted him to wear a tuxedo. He had never been to the opera and didn't own the right kind of tuxedo. He had actually never done anything like that in his life. He called us and asked us what he should do. We advised him that the opera could be a lot of fun, especially if this woman had so much appetite. We told him that this might be his chance of a lifetime to experience splendor.

He decided to go for it. He got the last available tickets to the opera. He rented a tuxedo, borrowed his sister's fancy car, and got a friend to drive them. He even bought her a corsage that she had not asked for.

She was not thrilled with any of it. The car was not a real limousine. The opera tickets were too far up. Needless to say, he felt like a failure. As a result, the more wrong she found his efforts, the less attractive she became to him. He just wanted to take her home and never see her or smell her (her breath suddenly repulsed him) again.

She could have been delighted that he found the tickets. She could have been thrilled with the car and the flowers and the fact that he wore a tuxedo for her. If she had appreciated his efforts, there's no doubt that he would have made another date with her, with better tickets and perhaps even a real limousine. If you don't appreciate what you have, you probably won't appreciate what you may get in the future.

This book is about sensual gratification and the ways in which it can make your life happier. Of course, sensual gratification is not the only way to feel fulfilled, and a person who is sexually gratified doesn't automatically become a happier person afterward. However, sensual gratification is an important part of many happy lives. Anger is a barrier to sensual appreciation. An angry woman may not tell a man what pleasures her. As result, he "loses," because he has not produced what she wants. There's an unspoken deal between men and women: Men are supposed to make women happy. When a woman isn't happy, the man loses. The woman knows this, and she is unhappy so that he will also be unhappy. Then she becomes even unhappier and more depressed. This is, of course, a lose-lose game, yet it is one that many people play.

Ironically, the physiological symptoms of anger can mimic those of sensual excitement. Heart rate and breathing increase, the skin flushes and sweats, blood pressure rises, etc. The only signs anger lacks are a wet, engorged pussy or a hard cock. If you are unsure whether you're seeing anger or excitement in your partner, it is time to stop any sensual activity and talk. If you pass this "test," it will enable your partner to surrender to you more the next time you do him or her.

We have known many formerly very angry women who were able to stop being angry and create wonderful lives for themselves and the men who were willing to love them through it all. These women are considered by their friends, relatives, and acquaintances to be some of the happiest people they know. Anger is a force that can be directed inward, at oneself, as well as outward. Once we recognize our anger, whether it's internally or externally directed, we can begin to deal with it better. We can begin to notice what upsets us and notice how we set ourselves up to become upset. We can take responsibility for our anger. Once we've done this, our anger no longer controls us.

Societal prejudice against women has begun to diminish with industrialization and the dawn of the sexual and electronic revolutions. In most industrial nations, sexism is on the decline. It still exists, of course, so women are still angry. But there are many more aware people in the world today than there were in the past, and some men and women have truly learned to love and treat each other with dignity and respect.

## ∼ When Do I Get My Turn? ∼
### EMO's Benefits for Men

Although this book emphasizes female orgasm and gratifying a woman, we want to describe some of the benefits that men will obtain by reading further. These benefits include a turned-on lover who is more fun sexually, learning to use your hands as sex organs, having a place to express your love, getting to feel like a hero, and getting to live your life with enthusiasm. Men can also learn to orgasm much more intensely if they practice the information provided in later chapters.

Men who learn about EMOs always ask, "What's in it for me? What do I get out of doing a woman?" The answer that we give them first is, "a happy, gratified woman." As we've stated, there's nothing more important in a relationship than a thrilled and gratified female partner. If you learn and practice the techniques given in this book, you'll be able to gratify your partner during each encounter. As a secondary benefit, you'll also experience more intense orgasms.

Men also ask, "When do I get my turn?" It's your turn every time you get to use your hands for pleasure. In order to do someone really well, you have to take a lot of pleasure from the doing. The best way to touch a woman is to touch her in a way that feels good to your fingers. Your hands are very sensual and feel a lot of pleasure, so feel her as you'd feel velvet or silk, fabrics that make your hand feel wonderful. The more pleasure your hand experiences, the better doer you'll become.

If you learn to touch for pleasure, you won't feel that you have to be repaid for your hard work. Once women learn to get off through clitoral stimulation by their partners, they may, at least at first, lose interest in touching their partners' cocks. Women have been "underdone" for many generations, and their newfound ability to orgasm can be very consuming for them. It's also probable that some women didn't experience much pleasure when they touched cocks in the past. They may have done it to get guys off their backs or for political or other sorts of reasons. But be reassured: A woman who has been done well and gratified will want to please her man, too, and when she does touch your cock, she'll experience a lot more pleasure than she did in the past. In fact, a woman who comes well can experience orgasm in her own body while playing with a man's cock.

Learning to give EMOs also increases your enthusiasm—for sex, for women, for life. Women are attracted to men who are enthusiastic (a word with a Greek root that means "to be with God"). Women notice men whose "motors are humming," as we say, and they want those motors to hum for them as well. Males of most species, including humans, try to impress females so that females will choose them as mates. Some birds have to carry around ridiculously large and colorful feathers and tails to get a chance to mate.[8] In many species, the males fight each other to demonstrate their fitness to be chosen. Playing football or other athletic activities to impress the ladies is probably a human adaptation of this process. You don't have to play football or be the best fighter in our society to get the girl, however, or to have the girl choose you. Women just like to see enthusiasm in whatever you do, whether it is courting her or just polishing your car.

This leads us to our next point: Learning to give EMOs can help you feel like a hero. When men are in relationships, they're often asked to produce or get something that their women want. Usually, this choice boils down to getting it enthusiastically or getting it kicking and screaming. We think it's more fun to do things enthusiastically. This makes you feel like a hero instead of a wimp. Women have the power to inspire men to perform heroic acts. A man by himself, on the other hand, only does what he thinks he can do. Other men, such as coaches and bosses, may motivate him, but only in relation to women does he feel effortless inspiration. (It's not surprising that all the muses are female.) Feeling like a hero is great, and men feel like heroes when they please women.

Learning about EMOs can also help you express love. It feels great to be loved, but it feels even greater to love. Humans all have a great capacity to love, but men aren't able to express their love as easily as women, probably because of social and cultural differences in the way we are raised. Women can hug and kiss one another as well as children. If a man kisses other men, he may be considered gay; if he kisses and fondles children, he may be considered a pedophile. When a man finds a woman who allows him to express his love and be romantic, his life becomes enchanted. This has another benefit: When men act romantic, that can help women to expose their sensual, animal nature. When women expose this turn-on, it allows men to express their romantic side again. I have written my best love poems after I was turned on or had great sex. Either gender can begin this loving cycle.

Finally, learning to create EMOs with your partner benefits you because it strengthens your relationship, and research has shown that men who are married or in a relationship live quite a few years longer than their unmarried brothers. Although some bachelors might disagree, we think that a man by himself is very dull. A man who is able to relate and produce for a woman feels that he's found a great reason to live. He feels useful and productive. He feels valuable. He feels like a hero when he produces something that he didn't think he could produce.

The ultimate functions of a male are to service the female and to keep the species viable. Human males have developed many ways to be useful to human females. Anything that aids a woman as she creates and reproduces life is useful, but such assistance can be separated into three categories: sexual gratification, food and shelter, and luxuries. Sexual gratification includes all kinds of attention and romance. Patricia Taylor, writing in *The Enchantment of Opposites,* calls these categories "attention, necessities, and extras." Women want gratification in all three areas, but the most important one is attention. If she's not gratified here, she won't be happy no matter how many extras she gets.

Humans aren't the only species in which males give gifts to females. According to Richard Dawkins' book *Climbing Mount Improbable,* among some species of spiders in which males are small and females are large, males bring females gifts of insects wound in silk threads. While she's busy unwrapping her gift, the male spider quickly inseminates her. Among many species of arachnids, females devour the males after sex, so there's no cuddling or smoking cigarettes after the act is completed.

We've known a number of women who stated that they wanted great relationships with men. But they didn't believe that men really wanted to give and please women to the best of their abilities. Therefore, the women didn't express their desires to the men with whom they tried to have relationships. The women hoped that the men could fulfill their desires on their own, via some telepathic magic, but the men only felt underused and unproductive. Eventually, another woman came along who saw the man's potential. She had enough confidence in her own attractiveness to know that the man could and would want to gratify her desires. The man had no choice but to go to the woman who had most use for him.

A woman who doubts a man's ability to produce for her actually doubts her own attractiveness. When a woman asks a man to do or get something for her, his first response might not sound like a testament to her wonderfulness. He might grumble or even say, "There's no way I can do that." She shouldn't take this personally or perceive it as rejection. Men doubt their ability to produce, and the grumbling sound is actually the sound of the man switching on his motor. He is already thinking of and planning possible ways to fulfill her request. All a woman has to do is to show confidence in the man and not get angry because of his grumbling or his attitude. She soon will have her desires fulfilled. It is in men's nature to want to please women.

We are not saying that women cannot produce for themselves or that men can't be as attractive as women. We are saying, however, that one of the best relationships between men and women is one in which the man feels productive and the woman feels attractive. Some of the information we've provided in this chapter is quite general, but we believe it's useful in understanding why men and women behave differently. Not everyone exactly fits these descriptions, so if your own behavior differs from what we've described, don't be concerned.

# CHAPTER 5

# Know Your Body

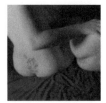

*K*nowing your body—and your partner's body—is an essential part of learning to have and create EMOs. Thus, this chapter starts off with what we consider the most underrated part of the human anatomy: the clitoris. You'll learn about its function, anatomy, and importance, as well as its size and how it engorges. You'll also learn about its "magic spot." There are other magic spots, too, such as the G spot, and we describe them and how to touch them as well.

We then describe the similarities between the bodies of men and women. Finally, this chapter closes with some essential sensuality exercises—one of the most important parts of this book—that help you learn about, turn on, and love your own body.

## ✒ Clitorology ✒

The clitoris is here to have a good time. It is the center of all orgasm (in spite of what Dr. Freud thought). Its only function is to experience exquisitely pleasurable sensations. The only other organ whose sole function is pleasure is the male nipple, and they are not in the same league. More nerves fill the clitoris than fill the head of the penis: approximately eight thousand nerves, about twice as many as the penis has.[9] This is particularly amazing given that the clitoris's only function is pleasure, while the penis has other functions: urination and impregnation. About fifteen thousand nerve fibers, all told, service a woman's pelvis.

Like the penis, the clitoris engorges with blood upon proper stimulation (see Figures 1 and 2). Unlike the penis, however, the clitoris does not have compressible veins that prevent the outflow of blood. Because the blood is free to leave, the clitoris doesn't get as hard as the penis for an extended time, but instead goes from hard to soft and back to hard, over and over again. When a trained woman is stimulated, her clitoris can stay engorged for hours, although its hardness may vary from moment to moment. According to Kermit E. Krantz's essay on clitoral anatomy in *The Classic Clitoris*, there may be a relationship between engorgement and the lowering of the threshold for nervous discharge, which means that it is easier to have an orgasm when the clitoris is engorged.[10]

A large clitoris isn't necessary for a great orgasm or proof that a woman has great ones. Depending on how sexually eager a woman feels, how well her clitoris is touched, and how confident she is in her sexuality, her clitoris can engorge to more than twice its unengorged size.

In a fetus, the clitoris grows for the first twenty-seven weeks of gestation. After birth, it grows in proportion to each individual's body. The clitoris does not seem to be affected by estrogen or menopause, although pregnancy may induce permanent enlargement of the organ.

The clitoris consists of three distinct parts (which may not seem so distinct, depending on the individual woman). The **glans**, or head, is the

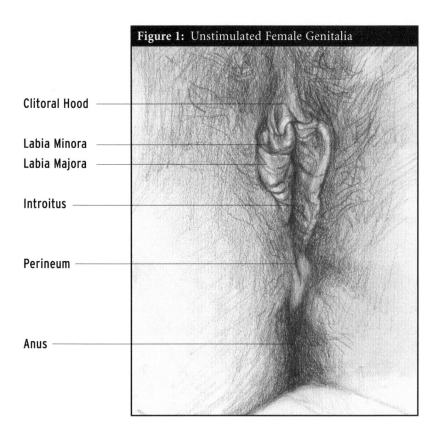

**Figure 1:** Unstimulated Female Genitalia

Clitoral Hood

Labia Minora

Labia Majora

Introitus

Perineum

Anus

most visible part. *Glans* refers to tissue that can swell or harden, and it's not to be confused with *glands,* which are tissues that secrete. Although the glans is most visible, it can be—and often is—hidden under a hood formed by an extension of a woman's inner labia. Most women's hoods are retractable: In other words, the glans can be exposed by pulling or pushing back the hood. Some women whom we've seen have their entire glans covered by a hood that

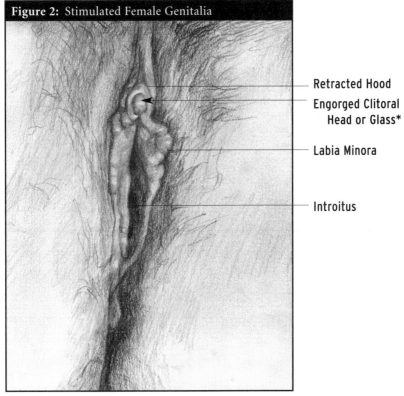

**Figure 2:** Stimulated Female Genitalia

Retracted Hood

Engorged Clitoral Head or Glass*

Labia Minora

Introitus

\* arrow pointing to "engorged clitoral head" shows most sensitive spot.

can't be pulled back. Other women have hoods that are only partly retractable. However, even those women are able to experience intense orgasm by being stimulated through their hoods.

The glans is attached to a **shaft**. The shaft may be slightly visible, but you're definitely able to feel it as it extends under the vulva up to the plates of the pelvic bone, called the pubic symphysis. The shaft has few nerve fibers but is loaded with blood vessels, so it also engorges. The shaft is attached to twin **crura**, or roots, which anchor the clitoris to the pubic symphysis. The crura subcutaneously arc out toward the thighs and obliquely toward the vagina.[11] They can be stimulated through the vagina and are actually responsible for the pleasure attributed to the G spot. In fact, they are the G spot.

There are no known specific diseases of the clitoris, although clitorises do have specific nerve endings for pain.[12] Some women with circulation problems may have difficulty engorging the clitoris, but we haven't seen this in any of our students or heard about any women who were unable to have an orgasm.

Very little research has been done on the clitoris. *Clitorology* is not in the dictionary. We hope that this wonderful organ, so poorly researched now, will become better understood and known in the near future. We've seen only one book exclusively devoted to it, in fact: *The Classic Clitoris* (see the Bibliography). Even this book, however, doesn't describe any methods or techniques for stimulating the clitoris. It even has a hard time explaining the derivation of the word *clitoris*, because prior research and literature is so limited. The book includes two interesting sections, one written in the 1950s on the clitoris's nerve and blood supply and a 19th-century anatomical description.[13] Otherwise, the book mostly discusses comparative anatomy of various animals. It notes that the clitoris is found on most female animals, especially mammals, though some reptiles and other organisms also have similar tissue.[14]

The most unique clitoris is that of the female spotted hyena. Her clitoris is huge. It's so large, in fact, that it's difficult to distinguish the males from the females. The females are also more aggressive than male hyenas. The hyena clitoris serves as a vagina: Newborns enter the world and are conceived through it. They have more testosterone than is normally found in the females of other species.

We have seen many sizes and shapes of human clitorises in our studies (although none as large as the spotted hyena's!). There is no "normal" kind. We have seen some that start out large but engorge only slightly, and others that are large and get still bigger when engorged. We've seen one woman who had a clitoris that looked as big as a thumb. We've seen others that start off tiny but engorge to a good size. Some small ones, given increased use and attention, seem to grow or at least are able to engorge more than they did at first. Again, size does not determine how much you can feel.

## From G to Shining C

The so-called G spot (or sacred spot, as it is known in tantric yoga) is really the underside or root of the clitoris and its nerves, which can be stimulated from inside the vagina.[15] But the G spot pales in comparison to the real magic spot: the upper left quadrant of the head of the clitoris as viewed from the perspective of the woman or at about 1:30 on the clock face if you are facing the woman. If you, the "doer," can find this spot on your first touch, you are on your way to producing a great orgasm. (*Note:* Throughout the text when we refer to a location on a quadrant, we are describing it from the perspective of the woman ... the left quadrant is on the woman's left, the right quadrant is on the woman's right. Where we use "clock face" descriptions, we are describing them from the partner's perspective, as if you are looking at a clock. So, 1:30 on a clock face from the partner's perspective is the upper left quadrant from the woman's perspective; 11:30 on the clock face from the partner's perspective is the upper right quadrant for the woman.)

When you're doing a woman, it's very beneficial to look at her genitals. Use your hands to separate her pubic hair for a better view. You'll also need to pull back the hood of her clitoris in order to touch this magic spot (see details on how to do that in Chapter 7, "How Do You Do?"). Once you've found her spot, you really don't have to touch it immediately. Tease her as much as is fun beforehand. Approach the spot, then back off. When you're ready to touch the clitoris, we recommend using lubricant.

We've found, in every female student that we've taught, that the upper left quadrant of the clitoral head is the most pleasurable spot to touch. Some women out there may be more sensitive on the right side of the clitoral head, or even the middle. Indeed, a study has been done on cadavers that found more nerve endings on one woman's labia than on her clitoris.[16] We have not encountered such women, however, so we believe that for most women, the upper left quadrant is the magic spot.

We hear many questions about the G spot. The G spot is one of several pleasurable areas that are inside the vagina but not on the surface of the vaginal wall. These places feel a lot of sensation when stroked, but because there are no nerve endings on the vaginal wall itself, some pressure is needed to trigger a response here. They can be stimulated by inserting a finger or fingers into the vagina and exerting a moderate amount of pressure. The G spot is up under the pubic area, where you can feel spongy tissue. Avoid the twelve o'clock position, for that is where the urethral canal runs. Rub a little left and right of center, at the eleven or one o'clock positions, fairly deeply, with the pads of your fingers facing upward.

Two spots that feel great to a woman who is in orgasm and open to insertion of your fingers are at the three and nine o'clock positions. These deep pockets on either side of the vagina feel wonderful to the touch, and they feel wonderful to the woman when you stroke them with a bit of pressure. This stimulates the sciatic nerves, and she can feel the touch down her legs to her toes. Another stimulating spot is down at the six o'clock position. Press down and toward yourself to stimulate the nerves from the anus. You can also put your fingers really deeply into the pocket at six o'clock, which stimulates nerves coming from the cauda equina, the end of the spinal cord.

There are a number of wonderful places to visit inside the vagina. You must enter the vagina only when invited in, however. When you're doing a woman, you will know when you're invited by the fact that your thumb or finger is almost sucked into the vagina. By rubbing and pleasurably stroking the head of the clitoris and the external parts of a woman's genitals, you increase the likelihood of being invited in. By keeping your thumb at the base of her introitus, the opening to the vagina, she can suck your thumb inside if she so desires, without you having to use much pressure. You can then press down with your thumb or even press up with the back of your thumb toward the G spot area. You can then switch from a thumb to one or two or even more fingers. You can rub on her clitoris from above and at the same time slowly massage the clitoral roots, or G spot, from inside. This sensation of being surrounded can feel exquisite.

## More Alike Than You Think:
### Similarities Between the Sexes

The **apex**, or the underside of the head of the penis, and the clitoris develop from the same embryonic tissue and are considered homologous. *Homologous* means "to be similar to," and it describes similar structures that share a common origin. The testes and ovaries are also homologous, as are the Fallopian tubes and seminal ducts, the vaginal wall and part of the scrotum, the inner labia and the shaft of the penis, and the labia and another part of the scrotum. It's been determined that only the uterus lacks a homologous organ in men.

Men and women are very similar to each other, a lot more similar than they are different. We have the same circulatory systems and a very similar nervous system. The only difference is in our sexual organs and our secondary sexual characteristics, and as shown above, even these are very similar. This helps to explain why many women don't have orgasms through intercourse. After all, would you expect a man to have an orgasm by having his scrotum rubbed? Most women who do have orgasms in intercourse have either a connection between the introitus (the vaginal opening) and the clitoris or a large clitoris that is touched by the penis as it moves in and out. It is also thought that the clitoris moves against its own hood as the penis thrusts in and out.[17] Some coital positions also help the woman to involve her clitoris, such as the woman being on top of the man or lying alongside him. Nonetheless, many women find it difficult or impossible to orgasm during intercourse.

The similarities between men and women make it clear that women are not, as some religions or societies would have us believe, inferior to men. They also make it clear that men as well as women can experience EMOs.

## ⟿ Sensuality Exercises ⟾

These exercises are vitally important to anyone who wishes to explore orgasm and pleasure. They can be a lot of fun to do and can bring you a lot of pleasure. If you know what you like, how and where you like to be touched, and what turns you on, and if you can love yourself and your body, it's a lot easier to have a wonderful, fun time with a partner. The following exercises have helped many people discover their likes and appreciate their own bodies.

It is best to do the following exercises in the sequence given, as they are much like a recipe's instructions and need to be performed in a certain order. You also need to do these exercises by yourself, not with a partner. However, the instructions given are intended only as a guide. They're provided in order to inspire you to be as creative and imaginative as you like. We love to hear about new ways that students invent to love themselves more.

There's no specific amount of time that you must spend on the exercises. Most students do them in about an hour, but some take more time. We recommend that you do all five exercises at one time in the order given, as each exercise benefits the next one.

You will get the most out of these exercises if you do them often, not just once. Each time, you can do them with a different emphasis and focus. Once you've learned your own body, you will have the greatest gift that you can give your partner: a turned-on body.

# 1. Visiting Dignitary

Many students find this first exercise the most difficult one to do. But this is the most important of all the exercises, and when done properly, it will enhance the experience of your other exercises.

Pretend that a visiting dignitary (anyone you choose, be it a famous actor or actress or the Queen of England) is coming to visit you. Choose a space— your bedroom, perhaps—and clean it up so that it looks nicer than it usually does. You don't want to spend all day or night cleaning, so clean up fairly quickly, spending less than thirty minutes on the task.

Your visiting dignitary, as it happens, has the same tastes and preferences that you do. In fact, this dignitary *is* you. We generally treat ourselves so shabbily that pretending to be a dignitary helps us to start treating ourselves better. Because you are a dignitary, you want to treat yourself like you are special and important and worthy, which you really are.

Into your cleaned-up room, bring something that is pleasurable for each sense. For taste, get your favorite ice cream or fruit, a piece of cheese or chocolate, or whatever you like. Also get something tasty to sip, like your favorite juice, a glass of good-tasting water, or a glass of wine (one glass, maximum). Bring something nice to smell, such as flowers, a scented candle, or incense. Put on some music that you like to please your sense of sound. You won't want to get up and down to change the music once you start, so if you use a radio, make sure it's set on a station you like, one that has very little talking between songs. It's probably best, in fact, to use a CD player that can play a number of discs in a row.

For your sense of touch, lay out a silk or velvet cloth or a smooth sculpture or whatever else you love to touch. For sight, choose a pretty picture, or use your flowers or candles for this sense, too; it's your choice. For conceptual thought—your sixth sense—you can use a magazine, porno tape, romance novel, or even your favorite fantasies.

You then find out that your visiting dignitary will not be able to make the engagement, so you get to use the space created for your own special pleasure.

## 2. *Visual Inventory*

Usually, when we look in the mirror to examine our bodies, we search for things that are wrong. Our hair is out of place, we are too fat in some area, or we have a zit. In this exercise, you'll look only for things that you like about yourself. As soon as you start approving of one part of yourself, you will find more parts attractive.

You can do this exercise best with a full-length mirror and a hand mirror. Look for parts of your body that you like, from the point of view of someone who's looking at you positively. Use the two mirrors to view places that you normally don't see, such as your anus, the backs of your ears, etc. Also, look at those places that you see often, but regard them with more approving eyes. You are a researcher, so take inventory of all the positive things about your body, all the things that you like, and be as imaginative as you can, using different angles and different viewpoints. Take your time and enjoy your body. You can take breaks at any time for a snack or whatever you want to do. The more you really like your body and appearance and are turned on by them, the more ability you'll have to turn on others. You will have sex appeal.

## 3. *Physical Inventory*

The visual inventory taught you to see and appreciate parts of your body in new ways. The physical inventory is similar: You'll explore all the ways that you like to be touched.

You can check out very light pressures and firm pressures, pinches, scratches, touches with the backs of the nails, or only touching your hair. Any way that you can think of to touch yourself is good. Touch yourself over your entire body. Notice what you like and what you don't like. If there is some touch that you don't like, use a different stroke. Check out the different extremes of touches that you can pleasurably experience. Notice, for example, the amount of pressure you can apply to the outside of your elbow as opposed to its inside. You will probably notice that different parts of your body like to be touched in different ways. This is your chance to find out.

Take as much time as you can on this exercise, as long as you are enjoying yourself. Take breaks to listen to the music or to gratify any of your other senses.

There is no right way to touch. Everyone has a different body and appreciates different touches. As the saying goes, "different strokes for different folks." The more carefully and frequently you do this exercise, the better you'll be able to teach someone else to touch you.

## *4. Focal Point*

Choose a "focal point" on your body, such as your inner elbow, a nipple, an inner thigh, or any other part that you like. Now rub your finger around that area in concentric circles that approach and retreat from the focal point without actually touching it. Use a fairly light and quick stroke.

You may feel that the focal point feels like it really wants to be touched. We call this "tumescing" the focal point. *Tumescence* means an increase in sexual tension (it's derived from a Latin root that means "to swell").

After tumescing an area, you can detumesce it (decrease its sexual tension) by rubbing through the area with a slow, deliberate, firm stroke. You can check out different focal points, too. The anus has more nerve endings than any other area of the body except the clitoris or penis. This area is taboo for some people, but if you decide to explore the anus, you will find it highly sensitive and potentially very pleasurable. If you do explore it, make sure that it and your finger are clean before you start. You can also compare the sensations of using and not using a lubricant on your finger.

# 5. *Masturbation for Pleasure*

The reason we do not call this exercise simply "masturbation" is that people usually masturbate just to relieve themselves of the tension or tumescence they feel. In this exercise, you are not supposed to go over the edge. The goal is to make each stroke feel exquisite, and you are not doing it to relieve yourself. We would like you to stay as relaxed as possible throughout the exercise. If you're a man, we prefer that you do not tense and squirt. If you must ejaculate, do it after you have declared your exercises over.

We recommend that you use Vaseline for this exercise. We like Vaseline because of its staying power: Once you apply it, you do not have to add any more. You may want to place a towel underneath your body, as Vaseline is unfriendly to sheets. If you do not like Vaseline on your skin, you can use any of the many other lubricants available. Most lubricants are water-soluble, however, so you will have to either reapply them often or add a little water to restore the desired effect.

## ~ FOR WOMEN ~

Choose your clitoris as your focal point. Tease yourself by touching your genitals all over, except your clitoris. Touch for the pleasure of touching. Approach the clitoris and then back off. Lightly stroke your pubic hair a few times.

For the next part of the exercise, you'll need lubricant. (If you don't like Vaseline, use whatever type you prefer. Abolene is similar to Vaseline and doesn't need reapplication.) You only need a little. Put some on your middle or index finger. Pull back your hood with your other hand and start stroking your clitoris for pleasure. You are being a researcher, so you want to check out different locations, speeds, and pressures of stroking. You can check out how using different fingers feels, or even use more than one finger. You can use up-down, left-right, or even circular strokes. You are exploring your body and your clitoris; it is up to you to find out what pleasures you.

Once you find a stroke that you like, continue doing it in a nice, even rhythm. As long as you are going up, continue to rub, using the same stroke. When you change the stroke, it will bring you down. Remember to relax and breathe naturally.

We recommend checking out a short, up-and-down stroke on the upper left side of the head of your clitoris. If you tense up, remind yourself to relax. We also recommend having a hand mirror nearby so that you can investigate the changes occurring to your genitals. Your clitoris and lips may become engorged and larger, and their coloration probably will change. Also check out touching other areas of your genitals, such as the inner lips and the introitus, which is the opening to the vagina. In some women, these can be highly sensitive to the touch.

Just before you go over the edge, or when you sense that the next stroke won't feel as good as the last, bring yourself down a little by changing the location, speed, or pressure of your stroke or by removing your hand from your clitoris altogether. Start rubbing again when you feel like it. This technique—going up, then going down slightly, and going up again—will increase the tumescence (sexual energy) in your body. This increased sexual energy is what produces great orgasms.

Peak yourself and take breaks as much as you want to. The only goal is to have fun and learn about your body. To learn more about peaking, check out the "Peaking" section of Chapter 7.

### ~ FOR MEN ~

Choose your penis as your focal point. Touch the rest of your genitals—scrotum, perineum, pubic hair, etc.—to tumesce yourself. Then narrow your focal point to your apex (the underside of the head of the cock, which is the most sensitive area).

Lubricate the entire cock, except the apex, with a small amount of Vaseline or whatever lubricant you prefer. Don't worry if you don't have an erection; a cock does not have to be hard to feel good when touched. After teasing yourself, go ahead and put some lubricant on your apex, too.

Using a steady stroke that you like, bring yourself up to the point at which a few more strokes will make you ejaculate. At this point, we want you to peak yourself, which means to bring yourself down just a bit. Do this by removing your hand from your penis or changing the pressure or speed of your stroke. If you are really close to going over, you can either squeeze the head of your cock or apply pressure under your scrotum in the area where your prostate and **hidden cock** are (the hidden cock is the part of the penis that is inside the body, which gets engorged with the external penis and can be felt from underneath the scrotum.

If your cock is not hard or you do not feel that you are close to ejaculating, do not get upset. The only purpose of touching yourself is to make each stroke feel good. As long as you do that, you're doing this exercise properly.

You can peak yourself at other times, too; it does not have to be done only just before you squirt. Then bring yourself up again with your favorite strokes. We recommend that you check out different types of strokes, especially slow, long, and light ones. Men are used to beating off by rubbing harder and faster. They tense up and then ejaculate. They are really missing most of the sensual experience.

Bring yourself up and down as many times as you like. There is no set amount of time that is right. We have known students who only masturbate for a few minutes and other students who kept peaking themselves for a couple of hours. Do whatever is right for you.

## 6. Connections

When we are born, our epidermis, which is our largest organ, is interconnected via our nervous system. In fact, the tactile sense is one of the first senses that develops in utero. Years of learning to turn off our bodies cause the channels of connections to atrophy. The nerves are still there, however, and can still be made to function. This final exercise has enabled many students to re-establish the sense of connected touch across the entire body. You can do this exercise while you are in the middle of the masturbation exercise described above.

As you masturbate for pleasurable effect, rub either the clitoris or a small area on the cock, such as the apex. This is your primary area. Once you have that area feeling good and turned on, you are ready to connect. With your other hand, rub another part of your body, which we will call the secondary area. Choose a nipple, a lip (either mouth or genital), or your anus, which are all erectile tissue. Or choose the inner thigh or another area that you like. Use a bit of lubricant on the secondary area, too.

Rub the two areas synchronously. Use the same speed and direction of stroke, rub the same size area, etc. After a while, remove your finger from the secondary area, holding it close. You can even continue moving it without touching the area. If you feel anything, that's a connection. Many people don't feel anything, or feel only a bit of sensation, the first time they try this exercise. If the exercise is done a few times, however, you'll start to feel more.

Put your finger back on the secondary area and rub the two areas simultaneously again. Now take your finger off the primary area, keeping it close and even moving your finger as if you were stroking right above your primary area. Notice whether there is any feeling. If not, put your finger back on the secondary area and try again. Keep doing this back-and-forth stroking between primary and secondary areas for as long as you enjoy it. You can also check out other secondary areas.

Take breaks whenever you like. Have a bite, a sip, and a smell, or take a deep breath and notice your body. The more frequently you do this connection exercise, the stronger your connections will be. Some of our students were able to build a connection between their clitorises and their introituses, and that enabled them to be more orgasmic during intercourse. Kissing, too, is even more enjoyable if you can connect your lips to your genitals.

These exercises are magnificent, and if you do them regularly, you will quickly learn to become more turned on, and you'll soon start to realize your sensual potential. If you cannot keep yourself from going over or ejaculating during these exercises, acknowledge that your exercises are over and have a blast.

We've found a lot of variation in how our students prefer to use these exercises. Sometimes students want to find their partners after these exercises are over in order to have more fun with all the tumescence that the exercises have produced. Others have spent all their tumescence and want to go to sleep right away. After the exercises, some students like to use firm pressure to bring themselves back down, applying their hands to their genitals and pressing down. Others like to eat to accomplish the same result. All of these methods are fine.

CHAPTER 6

## *The Art of Seduction*

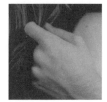

A friend of ours traveled to Rome after college. Some young women travel abroad seeking romantic adventures, but this wasn't true of her. She had led a fairly sheltered life and was not at all promiscuous. But she met a handsome, young, Italian man who charmed her into having dinner with him one evening. He picked her up in his sporty Alfa Romeo. She noticed that they were driving away from the center of the city, toward its outskirts. She became a little nervous and asked where they were going.

He told her that he was taking her to his home, where he would cook her a delicious meal. She panicked and said she thought they were only going to a restaurant. Before she finished her sentence, he had made a complete U-turn and told her he would take her back to the hotel. His willingness to turn on a dime for her and the possible loss of the evening changed her mind, and she agreed to have dinner with him at his home. They had a great time, including the best sex that she had ever had. She spent her next three weeks in Rome. She saw the man often, and he took her on tours to places that the average tourist never sees.

You have come a long way on your journey and have learned and maybe even practiced the sensuality exercises in the last chapter. Now that you know your own body better, you probably would like to explore someone else's body, and have them explore yours. You are almost ready to learn the specific techniques of "how to do." Before that, however, we would like you to understand and appreciate how you can seduce. The art of seduction is very similar to the art of doing. You must have your full attention on the person whom you wish to seduce or the person whom you wish to do. The better you become at seducing, the better "doer" you will be.

This chapter first discusses some of the reasons that people resist pleasure. Such resistance can be pleasurably overcome via seduction, so we next provide information about and techniques for seduction. We tell you how to create the perfect setting for a wonderful time and offer some techniques that help you hone that essential seduction skill: the kiss.

## Seduction for Pleasure

A goal is a hoped-for end result in a game, a problem, or a life. In a game, the goal is called winning. In problem-solving, it's called the solution. Once you've reached your goal, you can say that you have won your game or solved your problem.

In order to reach a goal, of course, you must overcome obstacles. The more obstacles you encounter and the larger those obstacles are, the more valuable your goal becomes. That's why we sing songs about "swimming the mighty ocean for her love" and "climbing the highest mountains for his love." We don't sing, "I'll walk across the street, if it's not raining, for her love." One key obstacle that people erect is resistance—they prevent you from gaining your goal. But this is all right, because if people said yes to all your offers, you would quickly lose interest. An occasional "no" makes things more interesting to you. We have known many men and women who stopped pursuing someone because their quarries were too easy. They always said yes to all offers, and consequently there was no game to be played.

Why do people say no? People say no to offers because they believe that they'll lose something if they say yes. This loss could be almost anything: time, money, self-image, etc. They might fear peer disapproval, or they might even say no just so you won't consider them too easy. Perhaps they lost when they said yes to a similar offer in the past, so they're wary about saying it again.

If someone resists a pleasurable offer that you have made, know that this fear of loss causes his or her refusal. It is not you (though it could be something about you). You can find out what this perceived loss is by asking them directly why they said no, or by asking questions that the person can answer by simply saying "yes" or "no." (For example, if they refuse a kiss, you can ask, "Is it my bad breath?" or "Do you have a cold?") By asking questions, you are putting attention on the resisting person. The word *question* comes from the Latin *questare,* whose root is "to quest." Overcoming someone's resistance is like going on a quest or an adventure. It's about reaching pleasure, and the best way to get to pleasure is by having pleasure now, by making the quest itself pleasurable for you.

Of course, it's also quite possible that the resistant person won't tell you what the problem is. You can then make overcoming their resistance a fun game. This is where the art of seduction comes in: You must pay enough attention to them to notice where they're at and decide which moves will best overcome their resistance. The good player's most important asset in this game is the ability to *enjoy* the other person's resistance. Once you've decided on a goal, have fun reaching it.

It is also important to continue in spite of doubts, be they doubts about whether it's worth the effort or doubts about why you are doing it. Just doubt your doubts. As all good salespeople know, all it takes to make a sale is one "yes," no matter how many "nos" preceded it.

When you seduce someone who resists, you must play with their resistance. Give them reasons to reject your offer that they have not thought of and then give them reasons why they should accept your offer. This strategy is called **push-pull,** and it enables you to have a lot of fun playing with someone's head as long as the goal is his or her pleasure.

Some people negatively judge the idea of playing with someone's head or manipulating a friend. If you feel that way, you should probably stop reading now and return this book. You probably don't have what it takes to give someone extreme pleasure. Or, alternately, you could read on, expand your viewpoints, and decide that manipulation for a good end is not a bad thing. It's actually a wonderful tool that can make the people you like feel more pleasure.

Being good at seduction means that you're good at keeping your attention on another person and being aware of their hopes and fears. This gives you a chance to gain intimacy and make them feel loved. Remember that resistance is only a reaction to feared loss. If you know this, you'll be able to enjoy the resistance and have fun with it, too. People really want to say yes when they're offered pleasure, and their resistance can actually make your goal more pleasurable to you. Resistance is a way that people use to limit their universe, and unless they are pressured to change it, they'll stick to the status quo and avoid taking risks or seeking new experiences.

Push-pull is a good technique for seducing women. Women love getting attention, and this makes sense, because they are the ones who do most of the attracting that's necessary in order to keep our species alive. Women love to be admired, pleasurably touched, given gifts, fed, and listened to. Sometimes, listening to a woman can mean backing off. Notice when a person has had enough attention and stop right before they notice that they've had enough. By pushing them away just before they want to stop, you make them want to come toward you. Pushing them farther away than they want to go makes them want to come back. If you pull on someone who wants to go away, that makes them want to go away all the more. A delicate touch is needed, however: If you push too hard, you run the risk of losing them. There is a fine line here, and the closer attention you pay to a person, the better you'll be at the game of seduction. The ability to determine whether a person is coming toward you or going away is also very useful later in the game, when you do their genitals.

Women, too, can use seduction to get past someone's resistance. They also have something that men don't have: **turn-on**, which is a trump card. Turn-on is the manifestation (or "womanifestation") of a woman's desire. Humans are mammals, and among mammals, the female, not the male, goes into heat. The male responds to this heat. Males (and other women) can be turned on by females, but they can't turn on females. Humans are different from other mammals in that women can go into heat at will, whenever they wish to have sex. We also have large brains, and this, combined with women's "volitional heat," means that women can attract both men and other women to fulfill their desires. (In Chapter 10, "Heat Cycles," you'll find a more extensive discussion of human heat cycles.) We don't consider turn-on a magical or mystical power, but instead our natural state. In order to *not* feel turned on, you have to non-confront that feeling. When a woman doesn't feel turned on, she has her attention elsewhere. Two ways to squelch turn-on are via anger and doubt.

When a woman does feel turned on and uses her turn-on to overcome a man's resistance, she can smash his resistance into little pieces, and any obstacles will miraculously disappear. A woman seduces a man with her desire. Some things can get in the way of her desire, however. She may feel angry toward men, or she may doubt her attractiveness. She must give up her anger, at least temporarily, if she wishes to turn on a man. Many women doubt their attractiveness, but in order to seduce a man, a woman must doubt her doubt and put her attention on manifesting (womanifesting) her desire. She must find herself beautiful and irresistible. A woman can primp, which means to take care of her body, with a bath, a massage, a pedicure or manicure, etc. She can put on clothes or lingerie that help her feel sexy and beautiful. Some men are conditioned to appreciate different parts of a woman's body, so if she knows what her man likes, she can use that information by wearing high heels or exposing her legs or cleavage. Whatever she does, it is most important that she likes and is turned on by *herself*, as it really does not make a whole lot of difference to the man once her turn-on is evident. A man cannot resist an irresistible woman.

People, by their very natures, enjoy pleasure. They want pleasure. Because we live in a society that worships pain, however, it's difficult for us to choose pleasure. We think we need special reasons and circumstances to seek and experience pleasure. Some people have special dates or times when it's okay to have sex or experience sensual pleasure. They might feel it's okay after a certain number of dates with a new partner, on an anniversary or a honeymoon, when they're in a foreign country, or when they're on vacation. Courses that we've taken and taught offered a great reason to choose pleasure: Assignments required daily orgasms, sometimes as many as three a day. We allowed ourselves pleasure in order to get a good grade or pass. Not doing the homework would have lowered our grades. By using seduction with your attention on pleasure, you can create and invent new reasons to choose pleasure.

Sometimes people will go for a foot rub or a neck rub, which are less charged than a genital rub. If a milder form of touch feels great, you might be able to get to an orgasm via a little more seduction. Remember, too, that doing someone is less charged than fucking or sucking, from which pregnancy or disease can result.

People choose pleasure if you give them a good enough reason to do so. Seduction is a fun game, and to enjoy it, you just have to decide what you want and then do what it takes to accomplish your goal. If resistances were too easy to overcome, after all, you wouldn't want to play, and if they were too difficult to overcome, you probably wouldn't want to play either. There is a large area between those two extremes, though, and that's where the fun is and where the game is worthwhile.

# *An Example*

It is wonderful when you and your partner are in agreement that a sensual experience, such as a do date, is something you both want at the same time. Sometimes, however, your partner needs a little more attention to say yes. Here's an example.

Ken loves to do Sara. Sara loves to get done. Sometimes, though, he offers to do Sara and she says no. She might say, "Later" or "Not now," which are other forms of "no." All these statements are forms of resistance.

Ken then makes a decision. He can get pissed at her because they are out of agreement and she's rejecting pleasure, but that is a sure way to lose. He can agree and pass on the do date, which is okay sometimes. But the best, most enjoyable response is to seduce her.

To do this, Ken has to get into agreement with her and then push her farther away than she wanted to go. He can say something like, "You are so right. We just had a great make-out yesterday, and it's probably too soon to have that much fun again. We probably shouldn't do it again until next week, when we will really want it."

At this point, Sara will probably feel pushed and want to come closer. Ken can then think up some reason that Sara hasn't thought of to explain why they shouldn't have sex. "You know, most people only have sex once a week. If we have it daily, you might feel like a sex addict."

Then Ken can take the other side. "We've never done what most people do, and you know you're not an addict. Pleasure is good for your health and your mind. We can have sex whenever we feel like it."

Then he can push her away again. "If we have sex too often, we won't appreciate it anymore. We will take it for granted and it won't feel special." Then he can say, "Actually, it seems the more we have sex and the more I do you, the more fun it is and the better your orgasm is. I will never take pleasure for granted, and I know you never will. Life is short. The only real time is now, and this will be the first do of the rest of our lives." If Ken continues in this manner, pushing and then pulling, pulling and then pushing, sooner or later Sara's resistance will start to crumble.

Ken, like any good seducer, knew before he started the game that people want pleasure if they can find a reason to say yes to it. Ken knows that Sara likes getting done. Putting lots of attention on Sara, or anyone else who's being seduced, makes the person feel attended to and wanted. (*Attend* and *attention* actually share a root, "stretching to.") The above game may work with Sara, but you must choose your own reasons for pushing and pulling by putting your attention on the person you wish to seduce.

## ᗗ The Setting ᗘ

Human beings, like many animals, create seductive settings in order to mate with the opposite sex. We don't advocate seduction in order to "get into someone's pants," however—seduction, to us, means knowing how to put pleasurable attention on someone you respect in order to give them a wonderful experience. Both men and women use various techniques and create pleasing settings to show the opposite sex that they are putting attention on them and learning what pleases them.

Although human males invest more than many animals in raising young, it's still females who invest the most, and females are therefore choosier about which males to mate with. She wants the best genes to mix with her own. Among humans, the "best" genes aren't necessarily those of the biggest and strongest man, but those of the man who can demonstrate his ability to care for a woman and their children. Big diamonds, fancy cars, and expensive restaurant meals are ways that men show their willingness to spend and put attention on women; so too are poetry, gifts of pretty flowers, and other ways that men demonstrate their artistic talents. This is not unique in nature. Male bowerbirds, for example, build immense artistic constructions with multicolored flowers, leaves, fungi, etc., to demonstrate that they are "good catches." Depending on the region, bowerbirds have different favorite colors and variations that are more or less valued by the female birds of that specific region. Male bowerbirds learn the rules of their regions from watching their elders.[18]

One of the first rules that human males learn is that women like to go out, be seen, and be complimented. Women have the capacity to receive lots of wonderful compliments, whereas men are often able to accept only small amounts of compliments. If you tell a man how wonderful and handsome he is more than a couple of times, he'll want you to stop. You can tell most women that they are beautiful and wonderful over and over again. Before you, as a man, make any offers or do any of the push-pull of seduction, it's a good idea to flatter a woman, to compliment her on her beauty, intelligence, and anything else that you genuinely appreciate about her.

You also need to discover her likes and dislikes. The more you know about her, the easier it is to produce pleasure. You don't have to go overboard with this (as Bill Murray did in the movie *Groundhog Day*), but do find out as much as you can. If you know her favorite food and drink, you can offer them to her. If you know her favorite flowers, music, scents, clothing, fantasies, etc., you can offer those as well. Find out her fears and desires. Women who wish to put their partners in the "effect" role also have to find out about their likes and dislikes and fears and desires.

Whether you're a man or a woman, let your partner know that you are there for them. Let them know that they need not worry about reciprocating, that you will take pleasure from giving them pleasure. Make it as safe and fun as you can. Also, remember to discuss any ground rules that are pertinent to the situation, such as using latex and whether there will be any exchange of bodily fluids.

Once you know your partner well enough, you can even set up a room for a sensual date, bringing along all their favorite things and topping the night off with the best orgasm of your partner's life. In our course, we call setting up a room this way the "Visiting Dignitary," which is also the name of an important self-exploration exercise. (See details on it in Chapter 5 and also check out ideas for setting up a room in Appendix B, "A Day of Pleasure and Attention.") Make sure that you like the stuff that you've prepared for your partner. For example, don't play country-western music if you don't enjoy it.

## ⤚ Kissing ⤙

We are almost at the part of the book where we describe how to produce an EMO. Before we get to that, however, we want to tease you a little more with some information about kissing. It is an example of how we are using seduction to get you ready for that big orgasm.

Like doing, kissing is a sensual art that can be learned and practiced. Many women will end a relationship before it gets very far if the man is a poor kisser. Many people work too hard at kissing and try to create an effect on the person whom they kiss. In most kisses you see on television and in movies, both parties are practically sucking each other's faces, with so much effort that it's a wonder they don't swallow each other. Sometimes it appears as if they are trying to stick their tongues down each other's throats.

The best kissing happens when you kiss in order to have your lips feel good, just as the most pleasurable way to touch another person is to make the touch feel pleasurable to you. The best way to accomplish this is to keep your lips soft and moist (but not too wet) and to feel with them. You can begin to learn to kiss while doing your "Connections" exercise, described in the previous chapter. Then, when you kiss someone, you'll be connected and feel the kiss throughout your body.

A kiss is a very full, sensual act, as you can engage all your senses in it. Besides touching, you can smell, taste, listen to, look at (you don't have to close your eyes), and even fantasize about your partner. It is a wonderful feeling to look at your partner as you kiss them and to take in their beauty with your eyes as well as your mouth. Vera is so beautiful from such a wonderful, close-up view.

There are different levels of kisses, according to where and whom you kiss. The most common kind is the perfunctory kiss. This is the kiss that you give to relatives. It's quick, with no lingering on the lips. Although this is the sort of kiss you'd give your grandma, you can also use it at the beginning and end of kisses that you give to lovers.

When you start to kiss someone for fun, rather than as a social gesture, you can begin with one of these small pecks, and then fully engage his or her lips.

You'll want to tilt your head so you won't bump noses. You can also hold the back of their head with your hand, as if to let them know that you want them. You can place your hands at the sides of their face, or anywhere on their body that feels good. Keep your lips soft, and kiss so that it feels wonderful to you.

You can move your lips around slowly and even tease different parts of their lips, as in the focal point exercise in the previous chapter. After a while, you can use your tongue, too, but don't jam it down their throats. You can touch their lips with your tongue and let it slightly enter their mouth, feeling the inside of their lips. If their tongue is there to meet yours, you can have fun touching your tongues together.

The best time to end the kiss is always right before they have had enough. You can always start again. It's sometimes nice to have one person be the kisser and the other the "kissee." When you are the "kissee," you can put practically all your attention on just feeling, moving your lips and tongue only if you are compelled to do so. You can exchange the roles of kissee and kisser. You can listen to your partner's breath, look into their eyes, and smell and taste their sweet lips.

If you don't like someone's breath, please correct it before kissing them. You can do this gently by first letting them know that they have a beautiful mouth and you'd like to kiss them, then saying that you really like a mouth to feel clean when you kiss it. You can them tell them that you'd really appreciate it if they took a breath mint or rinsed with some mouthwash. Once they do that, let them know that their breath smells great. If anything else interferes with your kiss, such as a tickly mustache or scratchy beard, make sure that you get your partner to fix that as well.

Kissing is a very intimate act, as you are face-to-face with your partner, touching and even penetrating each other, with the goal being pure pleasure. In many ways, it is even more intimate then genital-to-genital or hand-to-genital contact. We once knew a very liberated woman who didn't mind her boyfriend sleeping with or having all kinds of erotic sex with other women, but she would have killed him if she'd found out that he had kissed someone else.

The entire body is available to be kissed. Some women and men are very sensitive on their necks and ears, erotic areas that can be very enjoyable to have kissed. Some people, especially teenagers, suck or bite really hard on the neck to produce "hickeys." (This is more of a statement that the experience happened than one of pleasure, however.) There is a whole art to kissing a woman's hand—there is the formal kiss, in which you kiss the back of the hand above the knuckles, and there's the more flirtatious kiss in which you linger on the knuckles or even kiss the woman's palm and close her hand, which means an invitation to more. You don't have to add any sounds like "mwa" when you kiss. You can kiss a woman all the way up her arm. I enjoy kissing Vera's legs, especially her inner thighs. Cunnilingus (which we haven't discussed in this book) is also made more pleasurable by knowing how to kiss well. Just remember that the most important part of kissing well is kissing in order to make your mouth feel wonderful. The mouth is extremely sensual, and if you know how to kiss well, your relationship will be much more fun.

part **three**

*Play*

CHAPTER 7

## *How Do You Do?*

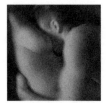

W e hope that you have enjoyed the ride so far. You are now ready to learn the specific techniques for creating intense pleasure for your partner. You don't have to master everything at once, so relax and enjoy every step of the continuing journey. After all, we are still learning new ways to pleasure each other, even though it's been twenty years since our first time.

People are not born knowing how to do each other, but, fortunately, they can learn the art of doing. Doing has nothing to do with intercourse—instead, it's the art of manipulating a woman's genitals, especially her clitoris, with the hands. (Doing can also mean manipulating a man's genitals, and we'll discuss that in this chapter as well.) We're not against intercourse or oral sex, and we believe that people's sex lives can include all aspects and varieties of sexual experience, but we do think that hand-to-genital manipulation is the most effective way to produce an EMO. Training to produce EMOs, which involves communication and doing techniques, also enhances other types of sexual acts. As we've said earlier, doing someone involves the seduction of his or her mind and total being, with the goal of giving your partner wonderful pleasure. Although you are doing your partner's genitals, your attention has to be on your partner, not just their genitals.

This chapter describes, in detail, how to do a woman and a man. We'll provide you with a general overview of the information and techniques that are necessary in this art: how to lubricate, how to expose the clitoris, how to position your touching hand, where to touch a woman, and what you can do with your free hand. After you've learned the basics, we'll describe some pleasurable techniques for doing a man. We'll also describe peaking, which can be used to intensify and elongate an orgasm, in detail, and explain the ways in which it's similar in men and women. Finally, we'll talk about the signs of orgasm and conclude with information on how to bring your partner down.

We have labeled this part of the book "Play" because it's here that we describe "doing" itself and give you the basic EMO techniques. However, the previous parts of this book—"Before Foreplay" and "Foreplay"—are equally important parts of an EMO, and so they're also about playing. We just had to play with your mind a bit first to prepare you to properly receive the information given in this section.

## ◅ Doing a Woman ▻

When doing a woman, one of the most important first steps is to ask her to get into a position in which you can do her. Basically, you want her to lie down while you lie down or sit next to her so that you have a good view of her genitals. Later, in the "Doing It Again" chapter, we provide a whole section about different positions that she can assume, but we'll give you the basic guidelines here.

Beds are a good place to lie down, but a mat on the floor or a blanket in the woods also works. You want her to be comfortable, and you must also be comfortable, because you both need to be able to stay in your positions as long as necessary. Also, in order for her to experience an EMO, her body must be very relaxed. Your body, as the "doer," also must be relaxed, because your partner will feel any tension that you experience. All your "doing" paraphernalia, such as lubricants, towels, and drinks, should be within arm's reach.

When you first do someone, it's a good idea to become familiar with her genitals. We've known students who had never looked at or had their genitals touched. They now realize how much they missed, and they're glad that they've finally learned. Before touching her genitals, you'll want to get a good view of them and notice and report what you see. (The "Training and Communication" chapter tells you more about what to say at this point.) This may mean using a fairly bright light, so that you can see what you are doing. A woman who is interested in having better orgasms values a man who is interested in looking and learning about her body.

Before putting on any lubricant, we recommend that you separate her labia minora (inner lips) with your hands, gently placing both your palms on her labia majora (outer lips) and slowly moving them apart. This separation gives you a better view of her clitoris and genitals. You can also separate the inner lips with a couple of fingers, pulling gently apart on both labia. Move all pubic hairs that might interfere with your strokes out of your way. If there are any loose hairs or foreign materials on her genitals, like toilet paper, remove them as well. It is fun to tease a woman's genitals before you put on any lubricant or do any stroking. You can lightly touch all around her genitals, except her clitoris, as long as it is pleasurable. This makes her desire you to touch her clitoris.

Some women may be so wet that you can use their natural lubricant. We think that it is even better to use additional lubricant, as the clitoral area does not produce much natural lubricant, and you may be rubbing for an extended time and do not wish to cause any abrasions.

You then want to expose the clitoris by pulling back its hood. It is a good idea to anchor her clitoris with the thumb of your doing hand, as the clitoris can be very elusive. On page 84, we describe in detail how to pull back the hood and anchor the clitoris. After you pull back the hood, stroke directly on the clitoris with either your middle or index finger. The entire head of the clitoris is very sensitive. As we have previously mentioned, the most sensitive part of the clitoral head is the woman's upper left quadrant or at approximately 1:30 on a clock face if you are facing the woman.

Now that you know where her "spot" is, you have to learn how to lubricate, how to anchor, and how to stroke for optimal pleasure.

## *Lubrication*

First, the lubrication. There are a number of different lubricants that you can use. Some are more viscous than others. Vaseline and Abolene are petroleum-based and quite thick. They have good staying power and need not be reapplied. They can stain the sheets, however, and some people don't like the feel. They should *not* be used with latex, as they cause it to break down. Many water-soluble lubricants come in different viscosities, too. We like to use KY Jelly, which is fairly thick for a water-soluble lubricant. It is also fun to spread on the genitals. If you are stroking for a while and her genitals start to feel dry and sticky, you can dip your finger into a little water, which causes the already applied lubricant to become slippery again. Some people like to use Astroglide, which is very liquid.

You can create your own style of applying the lubricant. Depending on which lubricant you prefer and how viscous it is, you can spread the lubricant with a delicious touch. When I use KY Jelly, I spread it slowly up from the perineum, along both lips. I use two or three fingers, and as I approach the clitoris, I spread my fingers apart and deliberately avoid lubricating the clitoris. Another method is to lubricate each inner lip separately, with a slow and deliberate touch. This is a good way to apply Vaseline. You can spend time on each lip, getting very close to the clitoris and then backing off. You can play with the area right under her clitoris, which is called the vestibule. You can even touch the clitoris from below, hold your finger there for a few seconds, and then return to the vestibule. You can invent all kinds of creative ways to spread the lubricant, and you can do it differently each time if you wish.

You need to keep two areas dry and free from lubricant: her clitoral hood and the thumb on your doing hand. This way, when you pull back the hood and anchor her clitoris, your thumb will not slip.

## Anchoring the Clitoris

The clitoris tends to move while you are trying to stroke it. This usually happens when you are doing someone for the first few times, and it is part of normal resistance. It sometimes happens even after you have done someone a number of times. Some women's clitorises tend to move more than others. The clitoris "dives" under the hood, back into her body, or even shifts from the left to the right side or vice versa. Anchoring the clitoris prevents it from moving.

To anchor it, first place the meaty part of the thumb of your doing hand against the left side of her hood (if you are right-handed) and press toward her clitoris, where the head and shaft meet. Then pull up on the hood, exposing the clitoris. If you are left-handed, place your left thumb against the right side of the hood and pull up on the hood to expose the clitoris. You are now free to stroke directly on the clitoris with either your middle or index finger; your thumb, exerting a light to moderate pressure against the shaft, will keep the clitoris from moving as it presses.

Some people have difficulty pulling up the hood to expose the clitoris. If this is the case, you can use your free hand to pull back the hood. Place your palm on the pubic area and press up till the clitoris is exposed. You can also ask your partner to put her fingers on her pubic area and pull up the hood herself.

## *The Stroke*

If you're stroking the upper left quadrant of the clitoral head, it's important that you use short strokes with your fingertip to produce the most intense sensation. Longer strokes, which we've seen many students use, tend to leave the spot and take the woman down. (It's okay to take her down, of course, but you want to do that deliberately.) Long strokes tend to travel over her hood or rub below her clitoris. This makes the woman doubt that the man knows where her spot is. Some women who have never been done before might like this type of stroke, because they can appreciate any attention given to their clitorises. When you do use a longer stroke, do it deliberately, and realize that it's not the best method for taking someone higher. If you're not sure what spot you are on, take a break and look.

People like to be touched in a myriad of ways. Some like light touches, and others like firm pressure. You can be sure that the pressure they desire will not always remain the same. Women who can get off really well have learned to do so with almost any pressure. It's a good idea to ask her what she likes. Some women don't know what they like, as they are inexperienced, and other women who do know still won't tell you. Some women even give you false information. You don't need to worry about this, however, if you touch her as if you were touching silk, velvet, or satin. When you touch these fabrics, you're not trying to make the cloth feel anything special. Instead, you are touching for the pleasure the fabric gives your hand. This way, you can feel sure that the touch feels good to her as well.

The best stroke for taking her up is short and on the upper left quadrant, with your thumb anchoring her clitoris. (See Figure 3.) We call this basic stroke the **bread-and-butter stroke**. Besides being short and on the spot, it is almost a pinching motion. The finger and thumb maintain constant contact with the clitoris and don't let it slip away. We describe the stroke as being like picking a $100 bill off a bar (or if you don't drink alcohol, a juice bar). The clitoris is between two fingers and thus can't easily hide. The "doing" finger can go to any part of the exposed clitoris and stroke with a repeated, dependable motion.

It is also important to "hook" your doing finger under the hood so you touch her clitoris with your fingertip, where you have the most sensation. The hooked finger can almost dig under the hood to reach the upper left part of the head. Right-handed doers: Tilt your wrist toward you, as if you are looking at your watch, so that you can easily stay on the left side of her clitoris. Left-handed doers: You'll actually have a better angle with your finger on the left side of the clitoris and your thumb anchoring on the right side.

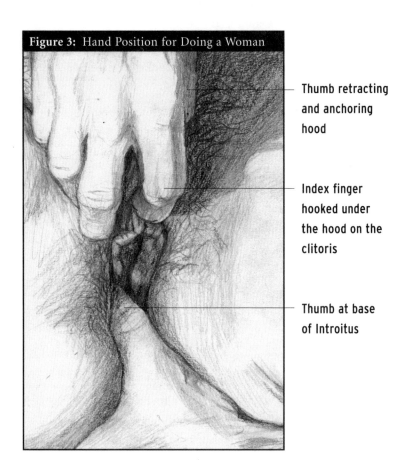

**Figure 3:** Hand Position for Doing a Woman

Thumb retracting and anchoring hood

Index finger hooked under the hood on the clitoris

Thumb at base of Introitus

Keep doing the exact same stroke, moving your doing finger up and down and up and down, as long as it feels good to your hand. Once the clitoris is engorged and totally exposed from beneath her hood, you can relax the anchoring thumb. All kinds of strokes over her entire clitoris will now gratify her, and she'll know that you know where her spot is. Although you've relaxed the anchoring thumb, she'll still like the feeling of your anchoring, so even though it may not be necessary for exposing and fixing the clitoris in place, you may want to leave your thumb there. You, the doer, can play with different speeds and different pressures on different peaks. Check out how she responds to a really fast stroke on one peak, and then use a really slow, up-and-down motion on another peak, barely moving at all. Play with a light stroke on one peak and a firm stroke on another. To extend the sensation of a peak, sometimes we recommend slowing down and lightening up gradually toward the peak's end. Remember to stroke for your own pleasure.

We recommend first learning the simple, short, up-and-down stroke, feeling in both directions. A number of other strokes also feel pleasurable, such as circular strokes, side-to-side strokes, and other strokes that you invent, but we feel that those strokes are best used after the clitoris is engorged and the woman is getting off well. That's because other strokes tend to touch her spot off and on. But be curious and explore her body, and you'll find many ways to pleasurably excite her.

## The Other Hand

If you aren't using your other hand to pull up the clitoral hood, it's free for you to use as you please. We recommend placing this hand below her buttocks, with two fingers on each cheek, making a V-shape with them. This position leaves your thumb directed upward. You can place the thumb flat against her perineum, with its tip snugly at the base of her introitus. This placement also gives you a good grip on her cheeks and help her surrender and relax into your hand. It also allows your thumb to feel any contractions that she experiences. You can also use the thumb to play with her labia and other parts of her genitals.

As we have previously mentioned, the best and only time to insert any fingers into her vagina is when she invites them in. You'll find that your thumb is suddenly sucked into her vagina. At this point, you can use your thumb or fingers for further vaginal stimulation (as described in the "From G to Shining C" section of Chapter 5). Inserting your fingers means, of course, that you have to give up their grip on her buttocks.

You'll want to continue stroking her clitoris while you stroke the inside of her vagina. The two hands stroking together can take her to wonderful peaks. Avoid her cervix, which is in the back of her vagina, and her urethral canal, which is up inside at the twelve o'clock position. You can use an in-and-out movement or press the pads of your fingers, with only slight movement, against the vaginal walls. Her vagina probably will be lubricated, so no further lubrication is necessary.

Here's a stroke that I like to use with my other hand: My two fingers (the index and middle) are spread, with their pads turned up, and I massage the clitoris from the inside by the so-called G spot, at eleven and one o'clock. The thumb of that hand is outside, above the clitoris, exposing and anchoring the clitoris so that my doing hand can reach it. Insertion can be a lot of fun, but the emphasis should still be on the clitoris.

You can also stimulate her anus with a finger, especially the little finger, when all your other fingers are in use. However, unless she has used an enema beforehand, don't move this finger from her anus to other areas, because the anus has many bacteria that could cause an infection. Some women also like to have their anuses stimulated from the inside with a finger. In this case, it's best to use lubricant. Ask questions, and proceed slowly and deliberately.

Sometimes, when I do Vera, there is no insertion at all. When we do an hour-long DEMO, there's no insertion during the first thirty minutes in order to demonstrate that insertion isn't necessary for a great orgasm.

## ⮞ Doing a Man ⮜

This book's main intention is to teach women to have—and men to give—great orgasms. Women have, after all, been getting men off since before the dawn of history. The world's "oldest profession" is about getting men off.

There's very little information about getting women off, so that's the emphasis of our book.

Nonetheless, many of the techniques that we have described above (under "Doing a Woman") can also be used to do a man. This section explores some fun ideas for doing a man. These include taking charge of his body, using light and slow strokes, touching a soft cock, playing with his hidden cock and scrotum, and cock sucking. We'll then give an example that will help you tie these techniques together.

## Taking Charge

A turned-on woman has few problems giving a man pleasure. The biggest problem she'll encounter, probably, is getting him to lie still and be total effect. A naked woman on a bed generally tends to resist at first, but once a man is naked on the bed, he is putty in your hands.

If you are doing a man, you have to let him know that you are in charge and let him know what you are doing. You can give him direct instructions, such as "Relax," "Stop moving your hips," etc. Sometimes a woman rubs a man for an extended time without communicating. He wonders if she knows what she is doing and when she will ejaculate him. It is very important to communicate to him that you have a plan and that when you are ready to have him ejaculate, you'll do so easily. Let him know that the goal isn't ejaculating in the future, but feeling the strokes that are occurring right now.

## Touching a Man

When doing a man, it's fun to tease him by lightly touching him around his cock. By touching his pubic hair, thighs, perineum, etc., you can get him aroused.

It's also very important to use a lubricant, whether it's Vaseline, a water-soluble lubricant, or even saliva. We recommend putting lubricant on the entire surface of his penis before starting to stroke.

You can erotically lubricate his cock, using a firm but light touch. Start from the back of the cock and end at its apex (the underside of the cock's head, which is usually his most sensitive area). You can also experiment with different ways of applying the lubricant and come up with your own style. Some men like you to warm the lubricant in your hands before applying it; other men prefer the coolness of the lubricant when it comes directly from the tube.

Just as when a man does a woman, a woman needs to touch a man with the purpose of having her hand feel pleasure. Stroking for an effect is usually much less pleasurable for your partner. Remember that if a man's cock is not hard, that does not mean he cannot feel pleasure. The nerve endings are still there, and if his penis is touched pleasurably, it can feel exquisite to him. However, if you "lose" because he is not hard, he definitely feels that, and the chances for his penis to become harder are doomed. So stroke with the intention of making your hand feel great. We recommend using the maximum surface area of your hand and fingers and touching your fingers to the area over his urethra. Use an up-and-down stroke over the shaft and head of the cock, and remember to feel it in both directions. You will probably want to lighten up as you go over the apex and head of his cock.

When men masturbate, they often rub themselves hard and fast, because their primary goal is to relieve their tension rather than to create pleasure. But he can and will feel more if you use a slow, long, light touch. You'll have to communicate what you are up to, of course. If this is the first time, or among the first times, that someone has rubbed him this way, it might not be entirely enjoyable to him, and you may want to mix in some peaks during which you use faster and harder strokes. Don't, however, give up on the light, slow strokes. Soon he'll appreciate those strokes even more than the hard, fast ones. Also try some long strokes, moving all the way down to the base of the cock and all the way up to its tip.

To take him higher, the technique of peaking (described later in this chapter) works with men as well. Stop stroking just before he is ready to go over, then take him for another peak. You will peak him by changing the stroke, just as men do when doing women. Any time you change the stroke, you bring him down. We have seen many women prematurely change the stroke, which kept their partners from going higher. It is very important to keep repeating the exact same stroke until you are ready to deliberately bring him down by peaking him. The stroke that best brings him up is consistent, dependable, and reliable.

Learn what he likes. You can have fun investigating the different strokes that pleasure him. You can give him short strokes just on his apex. You can use really long strokes, going to the base of his cock and pressing down against his body. You can use your other hand to play with his scrotum (it feels good to pull, tug, and push the scrotum, as long as you don't push it toward his body.) You can pleasurably touch his hidden cock, which is below his scrotum. You can use more pressure on his hidden cock and on the base of his cock as opposed to his apex, which is homologous to the clitoris and is where the highest concentrations of his nerve endings are. When you use a long stroke, remember to lighten up as you pass over his apex. You can lubricate his anus and play with that, too, if you both agree. The anus has the body's second-highest concentration of nerve endings, in both men and women. Once his cock is hard, you can move it around like a gearshift on a car, as long as you communicate and progress using small increments. Besides stroking, you can also hold his cock in your hand and play with different pressures. You can pull on his cock and use it in whatever way you like. Find out what his fantasies are. You can use those when doing him, if you so desire. The cock can be a really fun toy as long as you are touching it for your own pleasure. You can become an artist in doing a man and touch him in whatever way you create. If touched with pleasure, the cock will respond.

If he's ready to ejaculate but you're not ready for that, press the area between his scrotum and anus. This will prevent him from going over. Also try squeezing the head of his cock. If you've noticed early enough that he's going to come, simply remove your hand from his cock or change your stroke.

In tantric yoga, the man usually does not ejaculate at all. He's able to go higher and higher by using the technique of peaking. However, we don't believe that releasing ejaculate is harmful—semen is replenished quickly, and unless you're on a desert island without water, you can easily rehydrate yourself. We think that it's sometimes really fun to ejaculate, and other times it's really fun to go for more peaks and pass on this release.

Sometimes everything goes well when you do a man, but suddenly it doesn't feel so good to him anymore. The problem could be something as simple as a loose or out-of-place pubic hair that's interfering with a smooth stroke. Check the cock for pubic hairs or any other foreign materials that might be stuck to it or accidentally introduced when you lubricated him. Once, when a woman was doing me, it stopped feeling great. I asked her to lighten up, thinking that maybe she was using too much pressure, but we discovered that a loose pubic hair was causing the irritation. After its removal, she could use all sorts of different pressures that all felt wonderful.

You can do a man for a few strokes or a long time. You can finish him off quickly or extend his orgasm through peaking. You can let him leak pre-ejaculate fluid for a number of peaks (this happens when some ejaculate oozes out of his urethra, even cascading over his penis, but doesn't squirt in the fashion he may be used to). He may have contractions and be in orgasm throughout many peaks. Make sure he is relaxed, and don't let him tense up. Remind him to push out (see details on that in the next chapter) and relax, just as a man reminds a woman to relax. Only do him for as long as you feel like doing him.

If he has not ejaculated and wants to, but you don't want to go there, he can finish doing it himself. It is a lot of fun to ejaculate a penis, and many women can get off themselves and feel their pussies while doing it. Once men do start ejaculating, most men appreciate their partners lightening their touch. Of course, find out exactly what your partner prefers.

## Cock Sucking

Sucking a cock can be very pleasurable, too. Again, you have to do it so that it feels good to your lips and tongue, rather than for any effect. It's very erotic, and you can do him with your hands and suck his cock at the same time. Your communication depends mostly on what the man reports; if your guy doesn't talk much, you'll have to train him to talk more.

Although it's very erotic and potentially very pleasurable, sometimes women suck cock instead of doing, so they can avoid actually confronting his penis. They depend upon the act's eroticism and don't have to talk, ask questions, or put much attention on what they're doing. They don't have to see the cock, as it is, inside their mouths. Nonetheless, we think sucking is wonderful. It can be used to complement a do or as a separate act entirely.

## An Example

She takes him into the bedroom and tells him to take off his clothes. She takes her clothes off at the same time. She tells him to lie down and sits next to him with one leg over his abdomen. She touches his thighs and testicles and all around the base of his cock. She tells him to relax and that she is in charge of his cock.

She brushes all the hair away from his cock and just holds the cock in her hands for about a minute, squeezing gently on occasion, as it fills with blood. She puts on Vaseline, starting with the back and bottom of the cock and working her way toward the apex. She softly grabs his testicles with her left hand and starts stroking with her right hand, with a slow, long stroke of medium-to-light pressure from the base of the penis to its tip, lightening the stroke as she passes over the head of his penis. She feels the pleasure on her hand as she moves it up and back down again. She lets him know that she can feel his cock in her pussy as well as in her hand.

She continues to use the same stroke, taking him higher and higher. She then peaks him with a light, quicker stroke on his apex and returns to the slow, long stroke. As she tugs and moves his cock around in small circles, she tells him that she's having her way with his cock.

She plays with his hidden cock with her left hand as she continues to stroke with her right hand. He tells her that her naked thighs turn him on, and she tells him that she will rub them against his cock sometime. Then she tells him a fantasy about her thighs, which turns him on even more.

He asks her to squirt him, and she responds that *she* is in charge and will squirt him in her own good time. Just for that, she gives him another peak. She takes him on a few more peaks, taking him higher still. He's leaking, but she peaks him before he can ejaculate. Finally, she says that this time she is going to squirt him, and she deliciously strokes his cock from bottom to top, using both hands on it at once. He goes into stronger ejaculatory contractions as she slows down and lightens her stroke. She continues to rub until the sensation has been totally consumed.

## ✐ Peaking ✎

Peaking—which we've mentioned in the discussion above—is a technique that we use to extend and intensify an orgasm. You've learned where to rub and what pressures to use, but peaking is another secret that you can use to keep an orgasm going.

It's similar to the technique described in this book's "Art of Seduction" section: You back off or quit altogether before the person who's getting done—the "doee"—wants you to stop. Once this happens, they will be open to more rubbing and a longer orgasm, and you can start bringing them up again. We call this technique backing off and starting, or, more simply, peaking. Peaking is similar for men and women "doees," and peaking techniques can be used by both partners, unless we specifically say that the technique is intended for just one sex.

If you rub your partner without stopping, your partner either has a quick orgasm, begins to perceive your touch as painful, or stops feeling your touch altogether. Rubbing a person in the same way on the same area causes their nerves to go numb and stop firing. Then the person feels no more sensation. That's not something you want to happen, as your partner will trust you less and feel less inclined to repeat the experience. When peaking your partner, you stop or change the stroke just before they either go over or stop feeling. Peaking allows tumescence to build. Each time you peak your partner, it allows the energy to reach a higher level.

You can peak your partner via various techniques. Any time you change a rhythmic, steady stroke by introducing a different pressure or different speed or changing the area you stroke, you bring someone down. You can also deliberately bring someone down by using firm pressure, without moving. Perhaps the simplest way is to remove your hand from their body altogether. This can be done for a split second, a few seconds, or even a few minutes, depending on how you feel things are going. Then you can return to the old, steady, dependable stroke, and they will go back up. You do not want to change the stroke every few seconds. Your goal is to get them as high as you can. Another fun way to peak a woman is to bring her up with a short stroke on the clitoris and then peak her by dipping your finger down to her inner lips and introitus, lubricating your finger with her juices, and slowly bringing your finger back up to her clitoris. The most important part of bringing someone down is your intention. If you use your intention correctly, you can bring your partner down with almost the same stroke that you used to bring them up.

Changing or quitting the stroke just before your partner is ready to go down puts you in control of their orgasm. It also gives you a chance to take breaks, which is an essential part of doing. Some people think that they shouldn't take any breaks, that breaks spoil what's happening. This isn't true. Breaks are a great time to talk and ask questions, and they help you take your partner higher. Breaks give the participants a chance to feel more. As you get better and more experienced at doing, you'll naturally learn when and how long to break. There's no wrong time for a break; it's better to break too often than not often enough. "Newcomers" may need to take frequent or lengthy breaks, but experienced, advanced comers may not need to take many or have them last very long.

The length of time that you wait before bringing your partner back up depends on what you feel. There is no formula to fall back on. Sometimes, if the woman or man is getting off really well, you may only take a split-second break before continuing to bring them up. You can do this for a number of peaks, and as long as they respond to your touch with pleasure, there is no reason to lengthen the breaks. The peaks themselves (the length and intensity of the orgasm between breaks) can last from a couple strokes to a number of minutes, and the breaks can also be short or long. To know how long to wait, you have to pay attention and notice your partner's orgasmic intensity at all times.

Sometimes women are such "holdouts" that they wait till the last peak before they get off well. (In general, men don't resist as much.) You can tease her by saying that the peak you're giving her is the last one, and if she responds well to that, repeat that line on the next peak. Sometimes women wait till they think the touching is over before their defenses drop. At this point, you want to bring her up again, and this just might give her a higher peak than she'd bargained for. This "trick" has worked on more than one woman who really wanted to have a great orgasm but whose fears made her feel less. When you trick a woman into a great time, she will appreciate your art.

Knowing when to peak and when to start again are key ingredients in a great orgasm. But, you may wonder, how do you know when to peak your partner? To figure this out, you must first have confidence in yourself. Trust your feelings and pay attention. When your attention is fully upon your partner's orgasm and you have the integrity to trust your feelings, you'll know just the right time for a peak. Your attention will tell you if your partner is going up or down and will help you read their orgasm. People who are new at doing give a lot of attention to what they're doing, so they may not be fully aware of where their partner is and whether they need to be peaked. As people get better acquainted with doing, they get better at reading the orgasm. If you start to wonder whether you should take a break, always take at least a short one. It's better to peak too early than too late.

Talking while you're doing is a good way to help yourself read the orgasm. Say, "I can feel you going up," "You are still going up," "You are going higher," or "Your intensity is increasing." When you don't feel your partner responding to your words or going higher, you know it's time for a break.

Sensation also tells you when to peak. As you touch your partner's genitals, you feel the sensation in your finger and hands. If the sensation feels pleasurable and gets stronger, that means your partner is going up. If it feels less pleasurable, they're going down. Visual cues also help—for example, you can tell that a man is about to ejaculate when the head of his cock becomes bigger and more bulbous and turns a deeper red-purple color. This **secondary erection** occurs just a few seconds before take-off. Reading these sensory cues is one of the most difficult EMO techniques to master, but with a just a little practice, you'll become more adept at it.

When you find yourself wondering whether to peak your partner or stop rubbing, you've already missed your first opportunity to "quit" them before they quit you. Your attention has already moved from their orgasm into your head. This is normal for someone who's learning how to "do," and you shouldn't beat yourself up for it. Take a break and start talking. You can even tell your partner that you felt them going away and ask them what they were thinking about. This is a good question because there's a connection between your lapse of attention and what they experience. Regain control of this situation by getting into agreement with it and noting aloud that your partner has left. This way, you can regain their confidence. You must not blame your partner for going down. To fight them and try to get them to go up when they are going down is self-defeating. Again, all is not lost, and you can recover by getting into agreement with the situation and communicating what you feel to your partner.

Peaking—stopping right before your partner wants to stop—demonstrates to your partner that you have your attention on them and makes it easier for them to surrender their orgasm to you. As you become a better "doing" artist, peaking will become one of the many tools that help your partner have more intense orgasms (other techniques include talking, trusting and reporting your feelings, describing her body, relaxing, pushing out, attention, and intention). All of these tools can also help your partner have longer orgasms—you can help them feel and come on the first stroke and continue for many minutes or even hours.

Another way to lengthen an orgasm is to deliberately agree with your partner that you'll do them for a specific period of time that is longer than the period of their usual orgasm. (This technique is only useful if you're familiar with your partner and have frequently done them before.) If you usually do them for ten minutes, agree to do them for fifteen or twenty minutes. If that goes well, you can later try thirty or more minutes. When you have longer "dos," it's more important than ever to keeping communicating. Most of the time, Vera and I do each other for about fifteen minutes. Sometimes we do it longer—in our one-hour DEMOs, for example—and sometimes we only do it for a couple of minutes. It's a good idea, especially when you're first training, to keep the do on the short side. Some of our new students have had their partners rub on them for an hour or more. Unless they're great at communicating and taking lots of breaks, what probably happens during such sessions is that both the "doer" and "doee" space out and don't feel for a good part of that hour.

## ⤜ Signs of Orgasm ⤛

When a woman gets off really well, you feel it in the thumb of your hand by her introitus and in your doing finger. She has strong contractions by both her introitus and anus. These contractions are so numerous that they aren't countable.

She may experience **abdominal ridging**, which is similar to a wave of energy passing through her abdominal area. Her abdomen contracts and undulates in waves that can be small, quite extreme, or anything in between. Ridging is involuntary; it's part of the orgasm and shouldn't be interpreted as tensing or thrashing. Ejaculatory fluid may or may not come out of her vagina.

Your doing finger feels her sensation directly from her clitoris, which may even feel somewhat like electrical impulses. Sounds that might be described as moans may come from her throat. Her genital area, face, and neck are engorged with blood. Her nipples may be aroused. She may glisten with perspiration. Her heart rate and breathing may increase. Her fingers and toes may spread. These are all signs of orgasm, and she will have some, if not all, of these signs. Men have many of these signs, too, including contractions in the penis and genital area and the release of ejaculatory fluid.

## ✎ Bringing Your Partner Down ✎

We have given you a lot of information on ways to bring your partner up (tumesce them) and extend the orgasm. It is also important to know how to bring someone down (detumesce them), as it is very pleasurable and helps them to function better after their sensual experience is over.

You bring someone down by intending them to come down. You also use a slower, firmer touch. Bring a woman down by placing your hand over her pubic bone and simply applying a bit of pressure. Bring a man down through firm pressure on his body: abdomen, chest, thighs, forehead, feet, almost anywhere except on his cock. Don't use much pressure at first; add more pressure slowly if your partner desires it. If you still feel contractions and sensations in your hand, there is orgasm that should be had on the down side as well as on the way up. At this point, you might want to peak them, bringing them up a bit with some stroking and then reapplying firm pressure to take them down another level. You can actually do quite a few peaks on the way down, although most people don't because they have a prejudice against "down" as opposed to "up." Some people just stop altogether after their partner is no longer going up—they're missing a fun part of the ride. Of course, nothing bad will happen to your partner if you have to quit before they come down all the way. After a person has had an EMO, they're able to function perfectly well, perhaps even better than usual. They are refreshed, look beautiful, glow, and feel glorious.

When bringing down someone who's had a tensed-up orgasm—a man who's ejaculated, for example—you'll find that they generally don't want their genitals touched at all afterward. The more relaxed their orgasm, the longer you can keep touching them.

A wonderful "bringing down" technique for women is the **pull-up** (see Figure 4). Insert your two middle fingers, both facing up, inside the vagina and under the pubic bone. Separate them so you don't squeeze the urethral canal, and then pull both fingers upward at the same time while you press the palm of your "doing" hand downward on her pubic bone. You can hold this position for a number of seconds, and some women have strong contractions as you do this. Only insert your fingers if your partner agrees to it, however.

After bringing your partner down to a functional level, you can end the orgasm with a wonderful toweling off. We like to use soft washcloths. Fold them in half and then, starting from the perineum, slowly bring the cloth up, using moderate to firm pressure (depending on what pressure your partner prefers). Pass the cloth over the inner lips and finally over the clitoris and its

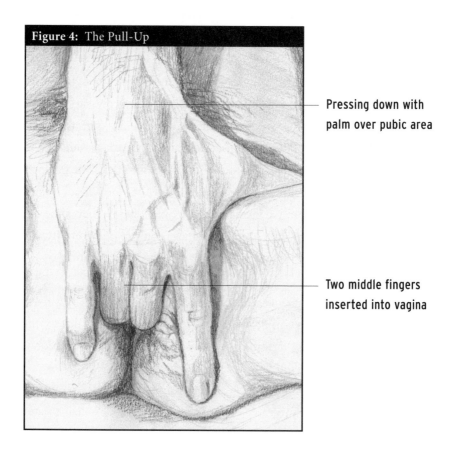

**Figure 4:** The Pull-Up

Pressing down with palm over pubic area

Two middle fingers inserted into vagina

hood. She will probably have some more contractions, especially when you go over the clitoris. The clitoris has probably now gone back under the hood and become less engorged. Wipe off all the excess lubricant or ejaculate. We have known some people who like to use warm water on the washcloth first and then use a second dry one. This is not necessary, but it can be fun, too.

You can towel men off as well. Most men to whom we've talked prefer that women dab the towel on their cock after they've ejaculated, rather than rubbing the towel as on a woman's genitals.

The extent to which you bring someone down after a do depends on who it is and what they will be doing next. If you do someone who has to go to work immediately afterward, it's a good idea to bring them down all the way. Some women like to stay up there after being done, and if she's not operating any heavy machinery or driving a car, let that choice be hers and just towel her off. Sometimes she might want to come down by having intercourse (the time just after a do is great for intercourse), or she might not want to come down until she does you. Eating is another way to come down—after a great orgasm, food tastes better than ever.

We have just gone through quite a few important EMO techniques. Incorporate as many of them as you can into your practice, and remember that you will probably have to reread some of the sections as you learn how to position your hands and exactly how to do your partner. The more you do, the more natural these techniques will become. In the next chapter, we will discuss how to "train" your partner and reveal communication techniques that will help you enhance your sensual experience.

CHAPTER 8

# *Training and Communication*

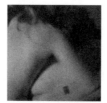

Vera, who grew up in Belgrade and Saltzburg and moved to New York City when she was sixteen, got married for the first time at age twenty (to an actor). Her grandmother—the first woman lawyer in Serbia—presented her with a book for a wedding present: *How to Train a Poodle.* Her grandmother had poodles for most of her life, but neither Vera nor her husband had a poodle, or any kind of dog at all. Yet the book had a lesson to teach: Whether you want to train a dog or a lover, it's best to communicate clearly, reward good behavior, and never be cross when you want them to do something.

Training your lover and yourself is an essential part of learning to have EMOs. We have just described how to do. We are now ready to describe some training and communication tools that are essential to doing. These include training from both cause and effect, the art of getting done, reporting what you notice, acknowledging the good stuff, and giving direct instructions. We also provide some techniques that will aid you in doing a novice.

Communication is essential because each couple must decide for themselves who will get done and who will do. Sometimes, when you have enough time, it's fun to play both parts. On the other hand, you don't have to reciprocate every time you get done. We know many couples in which the man does the woman (especially when she's first training) much more often than she does him. Sometimes the woman doesn't do the man but instead has intercourse with him after she's been done for a while and is fully engorged. Pleasure is available in both roles.

## ⤙ Training from Cause ⤚

Earlier in this book, you learned to train your own body through sensuality exercises. Now you're ready to learn about training someone else. This section gives you some techniques that have worked successfully for many of our students. They include helping your partner feel safe and cared for and asking them questions that they do not have to think too hard about in order to answer. The goal of both techniques is to learn more about how and where your partner likes to be touched. These techniques are valid for both men and women. (If you haven't already read Chapter 3's discussion of cause and effect, you will want to review that chapter before trying these techniques.)

When you do someone, it's a good idea to help them feel as safe and tended as possible. As a doing artist, your ultimate goal is to have the "doee" surrender their nervous system into your hands. You reach this goal by controlling the environment in a way that enables them to relax and realize that they're in the hands of someone who can take care of any and all situations and surprises. You do this by communicating what you will do before you do it.

For example, before you touch your partner or take your hands away from their body, you tell them what you plan to do. You tell them in advance that you will be responsible for any interruptions that arise, like ringing telephones or people knocking on the door. Let your partner know that you are there for them and that all they have to do is lie there and feel their bodies. Tell them that all they have to say is "yes" or "no" when you ask them a question. If they want anything, they should feel free to let you know.

In order to find out how your partner likes to be touched, you have to ask questions. Now, because you want to keep them at as close to total effect as you can, you want to keep your questions simple. A "yes" or "no" should be all the answer you require. Good questions include the following:

* *"Would you like more pressure?"*

* *"Would you like me to touch more to the left?"*

* *"Would you like it slower?"*

Don't ask multiple-choice or essay-type questions, because they make your partner think too much. In addition, your questions should produce "winning" answers. "Do you like this?" and "Does this feel good?" are not winning questions, because if the person says no, you might feel hurt. Your partner knows that, and so they might lie to preserve your feelings. Then things get sticky. Ask simple, winning questions so the person being done can stay at effect and easily answer you without worrying about your feelings.

Do not change your stroke until your partner says yes. Then proceed in small increments. You're building trust and don't want to do anything that might surprise or upset your partner. If, for example, you ask them if they want more pressure and they say yes, use a bit more pressure at first and ask them again if they want more pressure. If they say yes, add another increment of pressure and ask again. Once they've said no to this question, you can ask if they'd like less pressure. If they say no to that, you know that you are using the exact pressure that they want at that time. Keep asking questions until you find their desired stroke.

Once you have gotten the exact pressure, you can go on to ask about the exact speed, location, and length of the stroke, again using small increments. This teaches you how your partner likes to be stroked. During a doing session, a person will want to be touched in different ways at different times. So although you may have found the perfect pressure, location, and speed at one point, this does not mean your partner won't want you to change the stroke later. Continue to ask questions throughout the session.

Sometimes, you might ask your partner a yes-or-no question and find that they're unsure if they want you to alter your stroke. This happens more often when you're doing someone who hasn't been done often, but it can happen with anyone. Just continue with your stroke and ask another question.

It's a good idea to agree beforehand on how long the training session will last. You can agree upon ten or fifteen minutes, or perhaps the length of a certain piece of music. When the time has elapsed, let your partner know that the session is over. If you both agree to extend the time, that's fine also.

You can choose less charged areas than the genitals to train with at first. This is a good way for people who have difficulty talking explicitly about sex to get used to expressing themselves. Have your partner describe the area and boundary that they would like to have stroked. An example could be a left inner thigh from the knee to one inch below the pubic hair. You still ask the same questions, using small increments of change. Remember to inform your partner when you are going to put your hand on them and when you are going to take your hand away, along with any other information that will help them feel taken care of.

Once you know your partner and have become experienced at doing, you will no longer have to constantly ask them questions. If, at any time, you *do* feel like asking them a question, go ahead. Although you may not ask as many questions in the future, you still want to keep the communication lines open. You should also continue to tell them what you will do before you do it, so that they'll feel safe, and tell them that you'll take care of outside distractions like the phone. And, as a doing artist, you'll also continue to acknowledge all pleasurable feelings and describe signs of orgasm and your and your partner's turn-ons.

These deliberate training sessions are the best way that we know to help students find out how their partners like to be touched. After you've read through this section, read "Training from Effect," below—if you combine the directions given in these sections, you'll learn about your partner's body much more quickly.

## ↘ Training from Effect ↙

If you've spent some time doing your sensuality exercises and have learned how and where you like to be touched, and if you've found someone you'd like to have do you, it's easy to teach them to touch you just the way you like it. Here's a simple, straightforward method that we recommend to our students. This system works in all situations, not only in the bedroom, where you wish to teach, train, or instruct someone to do something for you.

The first step is to verbally approve of something that you enjoy about the person whom you wish to train. You could tell them, "You're wonderful" or "I really like doing things with you" or any positive statement about them and the situation that the two of you are currently experiencing.

The second step is to ask them to do something at which they can succeed. For example, ask, "Would you rub my left foot?" The third step is to acknowledge their efforts to respond to this request. Acknowledge them as soon as they've responded to you, no matter how small their effort, by saying, for example, "Your hands feel good."

Here's an example. You have agreed with your partner that you will be effect and they will be cause. As in the exercise above, it's a good idea to determine beforehand the amount of time that your session will last. Then you can begin the three-step training cycle:

*Step 1:* You begin the training by telling your partner something positive.

"I am so glad that you have agreed to rub on me."

*Step 2:* Then you ask your partner to do something specific.

"I'd love it if you would rub on my clitoris."

*Step 3:* Approve of their attempt to respond to your specific request.

Suppose that, after Step 2, you find that your partner is rubbing your belly button rather than your clitoris. You still go to Step 3 and find something good to say: "Thank you for touching me. I love doing this exercise with you."

Then you go back to Step 1 and find something to approve: "You have such a nice touch." Then you can ask them, "Will you please rub about six inches lower?" As soon as they head in that direction, let them know that they're succeeding by saying something like, "That feels really good; you have found my clitoris."

Suppose that now they're on your clitoris but are rubbing only its hood. Go to Step 1: "You follow my instructions really well. That feels great." Step 2: "Will you pull back my hood and rub directly on my clitoris?" Step 3: "That's wonderful."

You have to continue using the three steps until they are touching you exactly where and how you like to be touched. Step 1: "You touch me so well." Step 2: "I'd love it if you used some Vaseline on your finger." Step 3: "You used just the right amount. The sensation is wonderful. It is spreading down my legs." If you continue with the training, your partner will rub you exactly the way you want. It is up to you to make it happen.

Although this is a very effective method that works every time it's used correctly, many people still have a difficult time using it. The difficulty arises when people forget to include one of the steps of approval. Only give one instruction at a time. Don't ask to be rubbed faster and lighter or harder and to the left in the same breath. Each step is a separate sentence. For example, don't say, "That's great, and will you rub lighter?" Say, "That's great," and later, "Will you rub me lighter?" Later: "That's even better."

You may want to use extra steps of approval and acknowledgment, but each request is best proceeded and followed by at least one statement of approval. The more a person feels approved of, the more willing they are to follow the next instruction. If you like the way a person touches you and you don't want them to do anything differently, let them know that as well. Tell them, "It feels great," "Your hand knows just how to touch me," "Your finger on my clitoris is perfect," or "Keep doing that short, sweet stroke."

Before this exercise begins and the "cause" partner touches you, you can show them—using your own hands—how and where you like to be touched. Remember, however, to do all teaching within the "approval sandwich." That is, let them know that they are winning before and after you instruct them. Use as much communication as you need to help them understand. The person who wishes to communicate something is responsible for ensuring the communication gets across to his or her partner.

If both you and your partner know about training from cause and effect, you can do this exercise and the one above simultaneously. In either exercise, it's a good idea to practice the three-step training cycle described above, using a part of your body that feels less charged to you and moving to your genitals later. This allows couples to get used to talking about sex, and when they later reach the genitals, talking comes much more easily.

This three-step training technique works in all facets of life. You can use it to teach your children, get your employees to work better, or get your employer to treat you better. The world is really short of approval and acknowledgment, and when anyone adds this simple technique to their life, they are able to achieve more and make the lives of those around them more rewarding.

## What to Say

To be a great "doer" requires keeping as much of your action as possible in the present moment. This means that your mind must be clear. To be clear is analogous to an athlete being "in the zone." Your mind must be free of all extraneous thoughts. If you think about paying bills while doing someone, your attention is obviously not on their orgasm. If you think about what you will do next or judge how you're doing, you're out of the "zone." Really, thinking about anything other than your partner's orgasm and what you immediately feel while you are doing puts you "out of your mind."

Talking is a good way to keep your mind on what you are doing and keep yourself in the present moment. As long as you talk about what you're doing, what you're feeling, and what you notice about your partner, your attention is on your current actions. In some meditation retreats, participants must take a vow of silence. In the "Zen of doing," you must take a vow of communication.

When you're doing a woman, it's a turn-on to describe any changes that you, the doer, may notice, including the color or engorgement of her genitals:

✳ *"Your labia have turned a beautiful, shiny, purple-red color."*

✳ *"Your clitoris and labia have engorged to twice their initial size."*

✳ *"I can feel your clitoris getting bulbous and silky."*

✳ *"Your clitoris is sticking out from under the hood, looking beautiful and sexy."*

✳ *"I feel your clitoris getting hard under my finger."*

These statements are just examples, and as you start doing more often, you will come up with your own style and "snappy patter." Any flattery about how beautiful she is or how wonderful she smells is also a turn-on:

✳ *"Your face is glowing and is so beautiful."*

✳ *"Your radiance is captivating and exciting."*

✳ *"My hands feel so alive touching you."*

✳ *"I can feel you in my cock and you feel so great [only if that's true!]"*

✳ *"You are getting my cock hard; what are you fantasizing?"*

✳ *"Your pussy smells fantastic!"*

If you notice anything positive about her, it's a great idea to report it to her:

✳ *"I can see your female ejaculate oozing down your perineum."*

✳ *"Your contractions are getting more intense."*

✳ *"You are having strong abdominal ridging."*

Men don't care so much about being told how beautiful their penises look, but they do like to hear about how much their partners are turned on and how much fun their partners are having through touching their penises.

If you can encourage your partner to appreciate and acknowledge the pleasure they feel, using as specific a description as possible and without needing to think too hard, they'll open themselves up for even more pleasure. Reporting their pleasure and wonderful feelings also helps your partner keep their focus on the now, on their present sensation. Their acknowledgements are also a way for them to "swallow" the pleasure that they've just experienced before they take another bite of ecstasy. Meanwhile, you too can acknowledge all the pleasure you feel as you do them. Acknowledgement is missing, or at least underused, in our modern world, both in everyday life and in sexual life (where we have such difficulty in talking at all). Acknowledgement most benefits the person who does the acknowledging (although it's nice to be acknowledged as well). Because we don't often hear acknowledgement, we don't often offer it, and vice versa. If you are the "doee" and your partner doesn't care if you acknowledge, it will benefit you to offer as much positive acknowledgement as possible anyway.

Acknowledgement also helps you to avoid comparisons between past orgasms and the one you're currently experiencing. Making such comparisons traps you in the past, because your attention is on past experience rather than the present moment. But it's the present where you must remain in order to feel the most pleasure. It is okay to compare orgasms after your present one is over, but doing so while you are having one is certain to keep you from getting higher.

We've found that lots of acknowledgement and direct instructions usually take people higher. Tell your partner that you can feel lots of sensation in your finger and that you want them to feel even more. As soon as they go higher, let them know that you feel it as well. Tell them, "You feel great." Then you can tell them, "Take it even higher" or "That feels so good" or "You respond so well to instructions."

If you feel that they are tensing up, you can say, "Relax your body," "Relax into my hand," or "Push out and then relax." Just giving the instruction causes them to relax. Two instructions that we use with advanced comers are "Fill the room with your orgasm" and "Blast the back wall." You can let your partner know that they don't have to do anything other than listen to the instruction. The person being done does not have to exert any effort; they just have to listen, and their bodies usually respond by feeling more intensity and taking their orgasm to the next level. As we said earlier in the "Training from Cause" section, in addition to offering directions, it's always a good idea to report what you will do before you do it.

When you rub your partner's body, avoid saying things such as "Oops!" or "Whoops!" Even if you slipped up, pretend that it was deliberate, that you know what you are doing. This allows your partner to feel that they are in good hands. If they trust that you know what you are doing, they can put all their energy into feeling and their orgasm. Doubts about whether the doer knows what they are doing divert energy away from the orgasm into self-protection.

When our students have trouble because they bring bullshit into the bedroom with them, we tell them to leave it in a paper bag outside the room. When they're done with bedroom activity, they can always pick it up again, because they can be sure that no one's stolen it in the meantime. If you can't do this, you'll have to take care of whatever problems you have before learning to do EMOs. If, at any point during a sensual experience, you realize that you're "out of your mind," take a break and talk. Your partner's mind, more than likely, has gone somewhere else, too. If you can get back to present time before they do, they won't even know that you left and will appreciate that you got them to start feeling again so quickly.

You can see now how important communication is in creating and having great orgasms. To get the most out of a sensual experience, it's important to talk about it before, during, and after the do.

Before you start touching your partner, we recommend that you discuss what you are going to do. Arrange any time restrictions and discuss any limits your partner may have. Talk about how you will use direct instructions and what your partner does or does not have to do. This can be done very pleasurably and can be a turn-on.

Breaks are an opportunity to talk and check in with your partner in the midst of a sensual experience. How much you talk and what you talk about depend on the length of the break. If it is a short break, you might just say, "That was a great peak." If the break is a longer one, you can talk in detail about what you and your partner just felt. This could be a good time to evaluate and compare the orgasm, as opposed to doing that while you are stroking. Tell your partner what you plan to do next and how you expect them to respond. You can even tell them that you want them to quickly return to the point at which you just left them and to go higher from there. Find out if there is any special thing or stroke that they would like.

Talking about the do after it's over also adds to the experience. This is where specific acknowledgements are especially vital, as they give you something to remember and help you rekindle your feelings later. It's a good time to evaluate the orgasm and express gratitude for the experience. You can both talk about your favorite parts of the experience and find out if there's anything you can do next time to make it even better.

You can do someone with all kinds of fancy strokes and techniques. The best orgasms are produced, however, by uncomplicated, simple, and repeated strokes. If you feel that you have to get fancy and complicate your stroking, that is probably due to your partner's lack of feeling. If you realize instead that the only time that exists is the present, you'll keep your attention on what's happening now. By communicating what you notice, acknowledging, encouraging your partner to acknowledge, and giving direct instructions, you can use simple strokes, but the "do" will be far from simple.

## ⚡ Getting Done ⚡

Doing someone is an art, but receiving an EMO is an art as well. To feel as much as possible, you must be very relaxed. You must communicate your pleasure and surrender your nervous system into your partner's hands.

One of the most important skills of the "doee" is the ability to appreciate the uniqueness of their own body and sexual experience. We've seen lots of genitals in our work. They all look different. Everyone also seems to come differently. To think that you "lose" because your genitals look different than someone else's or because you come differently than someone else does is foolish and unrealistic. The best orgasm is the unique one that you yourself feel. Measuring yourself against someone else and using that person as your standard are sure ways to make yourself lose. The fact that someone else has a large clitoris or penis doesn't mean that they come well. If yours is tiny, that doesn't mean you can't come well either. You'll also lose if you measure your current orgasm against some past, fondly remembered orgasm. Each orgasm is different. In order to feel the most, you must put your attention on the pleasurable sensations you feel right now.

Remember that the sensation in your genitals is the most important thing to concentrate on. It's okay to moan and make noise when you come, but noise isn't the most important thing. We've known some women who carried on as if they were having the biggest orgasms ever, but the sensation they actually felt was minimal. The moaning that advanced comers do is done to enjoy that sensation in their throats, not to convince anyone that they are in orgasm.

After witnessing a woman demonstrate an EMO, many women respond that they themselves would like to have one. They wonder how long it will take them to be able to have one and how to go about doing it. There is no specific timetable: Some women are more orgasmic than others, and some women are more resistant than others. We've never met a woman who remained nonorgasmic after she had learned either to masturbate or get done. These techniques enable everyone to experience an orgasm, but only about 30 percent of women have any orgasms during intercourse, and even fewer women have orgasms every time they have intercourse.

If you're not orgasmic now or if you want to improve the orgasms you do have, the first step is to approve of whatever sensations and feelings you now have. Don't set a goal for yourself of some big, explosive orgasm at the end of a sensual act. The next step is to learn about your own body. The best ways that we know to achieve this are described in Chapter 5's "Sensuality Exercises" section. Once you know how and where you like to be touched, you can teach your partner or friend how to touch you.

Many of our women students worry that they will not be able to experience an EMO and are adverse to abandoning the tensed-up orgasms that they now have. Of course, we don't want anyone to give up anything. We hope that they'll add EMOs to their old ways of coming. But because being relaxed rather than tense feels different than a woman's usual orgasm, she may think at first that the intensity of her orgasms has decreased. If she senses this, we tell her not to give up and to try this new kind of orgasm again. We remind her to relax more and trust that her body will be able to feel without needing to tense. We also remind her that she needs to practice this new way of coming. Every student whom we've trained has been able to feel a lot more and to expand his or her orgasms once they've adjusted to a new way of coming. Once you realize the possibility of a longer, more intense orgasm, you'll automatically experience more sensation. Also, once you have taught your partner how and where you like to be touched, you can relax more.

Relaxing your body is one of the most important parts of achieving an EMO. When your body is tensed, blood flow to the genitals is constricted and less blood and oxygen are supplied to the nerves and muscles involved in your orgasm. **Pushing out** is a relaxation technique that has been successfully used by many women and even some men. Basically, it involves pushing out the sphincter muscles used in urination and defecation. Women can practice this technique by placing a small, clean, plastic bottle in their vaginas and then pushing it out. You need to push out for only a couple of seconds; then you can relax again. Make sure that you've gone to the bathroom before practicing this technique, as it can make you pee. Some people place a large towel under their buttocks just in case. Once you've gotten the knack of pushing out, your body will automatically relax as you do it. Any time that you feel tense, push out to relax.

Pushing out is also beneficial during intercourse. Usually, arousal causes the vaginal walls to balloon out, which tends to shorten the vagina. This can cause the penis to bang against the cervix, which is not only unpleasant but possibly painful. Pushing out prevents this, and it collapses the vaginal walls so that they touch the penis on all sides. This is a much nicer, snugger fit. The opening to the vagina also opens up, so it is not as tight around the penis.

Another essential "doee" skill is familiarity with the clitoris. Despite what Freud thought, all orgasms are clitoral. As we've said in previous chapters, we've found that the upper left quadrant is the most sensitive part of the clitoris. Once you're familiar with this "spot" as well as the rest of your clitoris, you can connect it to the rest of your body via the "Connections" exercise described in Chapter 5. This will enable you to experience a full-body orgasm. Some women describe EMOs as feeling like an electric current that enters the circuit of their bodies through their heads and leaves through their genitals, fingers, and toes; others say that they feel the orgasm originating in their clitoris and spreading outward from there, down their legs, up into their abdomen, and beyond.

Don't worry about how you're doing or how you compare to someone else. That will only make your orgasm decrease. The more attention that you focus upon simply feeling, the more you will feel. If fantasizing is pleasurable, that's okay. Verbally acknowledging pleasure is also helpful in taking you to the next level. Make your acknowledgements as specific as possible: "Your light stroke on my spot feels electric and spreads down to my toes" or "Your thumb on my introitus makes me feel surrounded."

As you practice, keep approving of whatever orgasms you experience and remember that your only goal is immediate pleasure. It's the same as trying to play Carnegie Hall: The only way to get there is to practice, practice, and practice. By doing yourself and getting done frequently, you'll expand your orgasms. We've known some women who, while training to experience an EMO, orgasmed close to ten times a day. (These women eventually learned to have EMOs so well that they literally changed the lives of people who witnessed them.) Of course, quantity alone won't make your orgasms more outstanding. You must have the desire to experience a great deal of pleasure, and it must become a priority in your life. The stroke that can produce an EMO in one woman might be completely ignored by another. It's the same stroke, yet one woman can fly to the moon with it, and the other can't even crawl. The true difference between the women is desire, willingness, and training. We've met other women who apparently orgasmed quite well yet were unable to feel it. Their bodies worked fine, but they weren't hooked up to their brains. After a bit of training, they were able to connect the two and experience sensational pleasure.

The higher the priority that you, as a woman or a man, give to pleasure, the more you will be able to feel. If, however, you see success as your ultimate goal in getting done or doing, you'll actually move farther away from pleasure. Orgasmic success comes with practice, but the goal of that practice must be immediate pleasure, not some great future orgasm. You will be successful if you go for the pleasure, but you may not feel the pleasure if you go for the success.

We've had students who liked sex and were able to have orgasms but found it difficult to give up control. They moved their bodies around, thrashed their hips when they got excited, and refused to surrender to their lovers. Any kind of sex is good, of course, but to achieve an EMO, you must surrender to the person doing you. If you don't trust the doer to do their job properly, it's up to you to teach them how to do you. You must also remain still and relaxed and allow the doer to do you. Each time you move, you demonstrate that you're trying to take back control, and that's not surrender. Remember that you really want to surrender. You are surrendering to your own pleasure, not surrendering to some person who will make you do things that you don't want to do. All the doer wants is to give you a great orgasm, but if you refuse to let go of the controls, they can't give you that pleasure. Being done puts you in a vulnerable place, but it is the only place where you can have more pleasure than you ever dreamed you could.

## ⁓ Doing a Novice ⁓

If you do someone who hasn't been done often or who hasn't trained his or her body with masturbation, you'll have to do your best in communicating and in creating a safe environment. First, find out as much as you can about how and where they like to be touched. Talk to them at length before you touch their bodies (especially their genitals). Let them know exactly what you'll do and what you expect them to do and feel.

Some people who have never been done before don't know what to expect. They may have doubts about how their body looks and works. Let them know that you find their body attractive, that you enjoy looking at it, and that you're sure you will enjoy touching it.

Before you touch them, tell them that you'll do them for only a short time—say, five to ten minutes. After that point, you'll both decide whether to continue or do something else. Tell them that you won't do anything they don't want you to do.

Mystery keeps us from focusing on pleasure, so get all the mystery out of the way via clear communication. Ask your partner about any fears they may have. If they express some fears, consider your partner "right" for having fears and do what it takes to alleviate them. Tell your partner that they are brave to explore something they've never done before.

Review the "Training from Cause" section found earlier in this chapter. You'll need this information because you will be asking your partner yes-or-no questions. Remind your partner that all they need to answer is "yes" or "no." If they want to speak more, they are, of course, free to do so, but they don't need to.

If you're a man, leave your pants on when you do her the first few times. This tells her that she doesn't have to reciprocate, take care of your orgasm, or worry about intercourse. Later, you can ask her whether she prefers that you take your pants off or leave them on. When you do someone with your pants on, make sure that your clothes are comfortable and not too stiff, since that might interfere with your attention.

Let your partner know what you are doing and proceed in small increments. A person being done for the first time, especially a woman, may feel only a couple of strokes and then space out, so pay attention. Take a break and keep talking about what you are doing. The break can last less than a second, or it can last longer if that feels right. Start again and continue with another short two- or three-stroke peak.

Once you have your partner at a place where they really feel those two strokes, you can add some additional strokes to lengthen their peak. If you add strokes slowly, you will be surprised by how fast things get. Remind your partner that there is no goal of future orgasm. All they have to do is feel their body and relax. Remember, you want to stop rubbing them before they quit feeling on the way up, and in many a female novice comer that means giving them only two strokes at a time. She might feel more than that, however, so pay attention.

Some "newcomers" are very excited when they first get done. Extreme excitement is an enemy to orgasm. You might think that excitement leads to orgasm, but it actually detracts from the feeling. Calm anticipation is a superior emotion to wild excitement. Often excitement gets stuck in the head, neck, or even stomach. This can diminish the pleasure that they could experience, so you have to channel that energy into their genitals.

Ask the newcomer to take a deep breath and relax to help them manage their excitement level. Sometimes, when we train someone new, I place my hand over her head and neck area and ask her to bring her energy downward. I slowly move my hand from above her throat to over her chest and then over her abdomen. Try this technique: You'll feel some heat coming from the area in which the energy is located. Let her know that you can feel the energy moving downward. If it gets stuck anywhere, remind her to bring it down a bit more. Once the energy is in her genitals, you can proceed with the "do."

Some women who are new to getting done have never had their clitorises directly touched. They may have touched themselves through their hoods, but they may be fearful of direct contact. If this is the case, it's best to proceed slowly. Put a big glob of lubricant on your finger and gently put it on her exposed clitoris. Let her know, of course, what you're doing at all times. Then touch the lubricant without touching the clitoris. Move your finger up, down, or around on the lubricant, still without touching the clitoris. Gradually get closer and closer until you are actually touching it. Stroke lightly and use the questions described above in "Training from Cause" to make sure that she does not want you to use a lighter touch. If you touch her this way gradually, she will feel safe and realize that it actually feels good to have her clitoris touched directly.

If you're doing a man for the first time, it's best to use the same questions. Once a man is naked in bed, however, he's less likely to resist than a woman. He might not know what to do, however, so you'll have to take control and let him know that you're in charge and what you want him to do (and not do).

Don't be afraid to touch a newcomer. Your partner will be able to tell if your touch is tentative. That will feel unpleasant, and such touches are difficult to surrender to. If you're unfamiliar with the genitals of the opposite sex, take the time, before stroking, to become visually familiar with them. Again, everyone has differently shaped and sized genitals. If you're doing someone for the first time, take the time to find out what's in front of you.

When you're doing a newcomer, it's extra-important to report any good feelings and sensations. The more you can report **specific frames** (descriptions of specific feelings or sensations at specific moments, reported in detail that differentiates these moments from others), the more you'll have to talk about later. Specific frames also add to the present experience and keep you and your partner in present time.

Resistance and relaxation are key issues when you're doing a newcomer. You may have noticed that we've repeatedly mentioned the importance of your partner's relaxation throughout their orgasm. If they tense up or thrash about, they resist feeling. It is difficult enough to maintain direct control and contact with a clitoris, and her thrashing makes it even more difficult. When women tense up, they are copying the usual male ejaculatory behavior. You need to explain relaxed EMOs to your partner and explain how her orgasm can become an extended, wavelike feeling, one that is far superior to her previous orgasms. When your partner struggles for control by moving or tensing her body, let her know that you are in charge and that you want her to lie there, relax her body, and feel your finger or hand.

If your partner continues to struggle, you should stop rubbing until her body relaxes. Sometimes, you can agree beforehand that moving, thrashing, and tensing can occur and are okay. Remember that we don't want you to stop doing anything—but don't expect it to be as much fun as it used to be. More doing and more self-training will enable your partner to have longer, more intense peaks. As your partner learns to surrender to you, they'll be able to go higher. This is why your communication and confidence are so important.

Be sure that you stop at the stipulated time and find out whether you should continue. If you're a good doer, you'll be able to stop just before that time, and your partner will probably want more. If you think they've had enough but they pretend to want more, it's best to quit. In future doing sessions, if your partner says they want more and asks you to continue, you can tell them that you'll rub for only a few strokes and if they don't go up, you won't continue. Follow through on your words. Usually, when you think they've had enough, they have.

As we have previously said, it is a great idea to talk about your experience after it is over. Many people have difficulty talking about sex, as we have been brought up not to talk about it. If you introduce the subject first and describe to your partner in detail what you felt during your experience, they will have an easier time talking about it. This is the time to bring up the specific frames that you described while you did them. If your specific frames are *really* specific, you may actually feel like those experiences are occurring again.

# CHAPTER 9

# Doing It Again

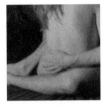

*T*his chapter gives you additional techniques to add to your bag of "doing" tricks. These include teasing, playfulness, curiosity, power games, dancing on the clitoris, and fantasy. We also describe the positions that we've discovered are best for doing someone. We provide some ideas on how to handle the "advanced doee," someone who already orgasms well. Finally, this "Play" section of the book concludes with some playful information on coming together.

Until you've learned the basic techniques of doing, those techniques will seem the most important part of EMOs. But once you have those techniques down pat, they won't be that important anymore, because fun will become the key ingredient. At that point, you'll create your own bag of tricks, because you'll have become an artist at doing and getting done.

## ☞ Fun First ☜

An old saying claims that sex is like pasta: When it's good it's really good, and when it's not so good it's still pretty good. This may be true for men having intercourse too, but we find it hard to believe that women would agree. Many women do not have orgasms with intercourse, and it can even be painful to them. In order to feel pleasure, to make love, to enjoy your partner, the key ingredient is fun. You can have fun when you're being done and doing whether you are an expert or a novice.

Having fun includes appreciating and acknowledging the pleasure that is occurring. Laughing and giggling are okay, but you should realize that they are also ways that people use to avoid the pleasure they feel. We are definitely for laughter, of course, and sometimes it's okay to ignore your orgasm if the laugh is good. But when some people begin to experience more intense orgasms than they have in the past, they laugh or even cry to escape the intensity.

**Teasing** is an important aspect of fun. Before you do any stroking, it is often a good idea to tease her genitals. Teasing is a good idea with both novices and advanced comers. Occasionally a woman may desire you to start directly and forego all teasing, either because of a time constraint or because she's turned on and ready. But that is unusual.

In teasing, you are basically using her clitoris as the focal point. You can lightly touch all parts of her genitals except the clitoris and touch other erogenous areas such as her thighs or nipples. Lightly touch her pubic hair with your palm or the back of your hand. Slowly press your knuckle against her introitus. Play with her inner lips. Touch the area above her clitoris, maybe pressing through the hood and teasing her clitoris with a little pressure, then releasing and repeating. She may be having contractions and other signs of orgasm as you tease her. Report all signs of orgasm. Take your time. Have fun; tell her that you may never get to her clitoris. This will make her want you to touch it.

As we stated earlier in the book, sometimes you may go directly to the clitoris, even skipping the genital lubrication and putting a little lubrication on your finger instead before you start to bring her up. But it's fun to tease her first and tease her again at any point in the "do" when you feel you want to make her come toward you. One good way to tease is to inform her that these will be the last few strokes or that you're going to stop any second. The difference between teasing and torture is that in teasing, you know that sooner or later you will get gratified. That's why it's considered a compliment when your partner tells you that "you are such a tease" when you're doing him or her.

The amount of teasing you should do depends on her response and how much fun it is, as well as any time constraints. It is best not to rely on any formulas, always tease in the same way, or say the same things every time. That's not as much fun.

Teasing, like any other technique, takes some time and practice to learn, but it will become second nature to you, and you won't have to wonder, "Which thumb do I put where?" You'll know what to do, when to do it, and what to say while you do it. Again, the goal is to have fun, not to feel performance pressure. You will feel more and more sensation as you practice, and your partner will, too. Once you're more sure of yourself and more adept at having and giving EMOs, you can experiment more.

Curiosity is a turn-on. You can be playful and curious even before you are an expert. Curiosity means being interested and attentive. It may come in the form of asking questions or through checking out new possibilities that turn on your partner. I always do Vera—and anyone else—with lots of enthusiasm, and I am open to finding new ways to tease and please. No two doings are exactly the same, and if you are looking for a formula that always works, you won't find it. It is best to go with your feelings and follow your bliss.

## ✒ Positions ✒

We have described in detail how to do a woman and have also provided information on how to do a man. Now we'll describe some body positions that we've discovered work best for doing. We've provided all the details, so that you can choose the one that works best for you.

Whenever you do someone, you want to assume a position in which you can comfortably stay for an extended amount of time. This requires lots of pillows and cushions. We have a dozen pillows of various sizes and shapes on our bed. It is a good idea to keep water in a glass with a straw nearby, so that you will not have to get up to fetch it. All lubricants, towels, and other accessories should be placed within a convenient arm's reach. If you like to get done or do with music, make sure that you have a stereo or boom box handy.

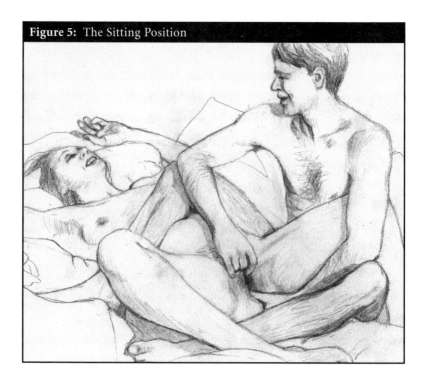

**Figure 5:** The Sitting Position

It is best to choose a position in which you can see your partner's genitals up close and in which you can also see their face—this way, communication can take place easily. You can accomplish both goals by either sitting up or lying on your side.

When you sit up, a number of positions are possible, depending on how formal you wish to be. In the most formal position, you sit in a chair, fully dressed, with your partner lying perpendicular to you at the edge of the bed. Alternately, sit at the head of the bed with your legs folded and your partner lying perpendicular to you. In our favorite sitting position, the doer sits up against pillows at the head of the bed, and the "doee" lies perpendicular (see Figure 5).

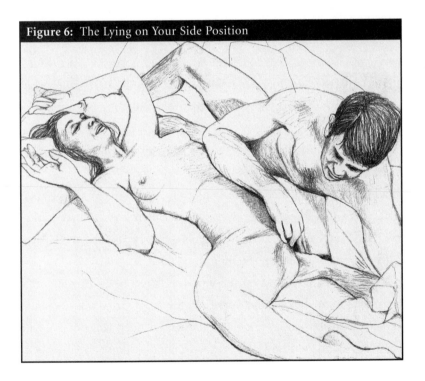

**Figure 6:** The Lying on Your Side Position

The leg closest to your partner's face is placed across their abdomen in a bent position. This leg helps your partner feel anchored and is also useful to you, because you can rest your elbow on the knee of the bent leg. The other leg is extended straight and placed under your partner's legs. In all of these positions, if you are right-handed, your partner's face should be on your right. If you are left-handed, their face should be on your left.

When doing a woman, make sure that her legs are spread and place pillows under her outside thigh and her head. Place your non-doing hand under her buttocks, with your thumb at the base of her introitus, and keep your doing hand free to stroke wherever you choose.

You can do someone lying on your side, too (see Figure 6). If you are right-handed, lie on your left side; if you are left-handed, lie on your right side. Your head should be on the opposite end from your partner's. First, put a pillow over your partner's inner leg and then lie on your side with your non-doing arm between your partner's legs. Rest on your forearm. Again, place your hand under your partner's buttocks. The side of your chest lies on the pillow on your partner's leg. Your doing hand is free to stroke. Add any pillows needed for extra comfort.

These above-mentioned positions are among the best for doing. They can be used to do a woman or a man. Many of our female friends like to use these techniques when doing men. Some women also like to sit cross-legged between a man's legs with his legs either over or under their legs. In this position, the woman has both hands free to play with his cock. She also can bend forward to put his cock in her mouth, if she should so desire.

A number of variations on these positions can be used; you are free to experiment to find the one that works best for you. Once you know your partner's genitals really well and are an experienced doer, you can do someone while lying next to them and stroking their genitals without visual contact. This position is nice because you can kiss your partner and look them in the eyes as you do them. It's a nice position to use when you first wake up in the morning or before you go to sleep at night, but you can do this only if you know what you are doing, and you shouldn't expect to get your partner as high as with the other positions.

## ✐ Playfulness ◟

Communication is an attribute of the good doer—you need to be able to communicate what you are doing and how you're enjoying the experience. Playfulness is another important attribute.

By "playfulness," we mean that when the doer does someone, the most important goal is having a great time. Playful doers use lots of teasing and seducing and overcome any resistance that comes their way. Playfulness does not mean that you grab or tickle your partner or make any sudden or unexpected moves. It does mean that you're enthusiastic and curious. If you can demonstrate your enthusiasm and curiosity, your partner will feel that you're enjoying yourself and that you're genuinely interested in pleasuring them. Your fun "rubs off" on your partner, so to speak, and allows them to have fun, too. If, on the other hand, you touch your partner and don't appear to have much fun, they'll shut down and feel less. The level of pleasure that you have and show strongly influences your partner. With confidence, intention and attention, enthusiasm, curiosity, and enjoyment, your partner will feel safe and appreciated enough to surrender their nervous system to you.

Here are some suggestions for introducing play into your "do." You can play with different pressures. You can use lots of lubricant, but then only let your fingers contact the lubricant, not your partner's skin. You can see how far you can feel pleasure with light pressure. You can go to the other extreme and grab the clitoris between your thumb and your index finger and squeeze hard. (When you do this, it's best to use the training cycle, asking, "Would you like more pressure?" and increasing the pressure in small increments.) You can also play with other erotic areas in this way. A man can take the woman's labia minora between his fingers and slowly pull them outward, always asking to make sure that he does not pull too far. Women can do the same with a man's genitals. She can try different pressures on his penis, from very light to hard, always using small increments and the training cycle. She can slowly pull his scrotum away from his body, just as he's done to her labia. Be creative and invent your own experiments to perform with your partner.

## Dancing on the Clitoris

Another fun technique that is widely appreciated is dancing on the clitoris and the pussy. This is a technique in which you can become quite creative. I often use music while I "dance" with my fingers. You can do and come to lots of styles and sounds. We sometimes use Brazilian and other Latin music with a nice beat. Vera likes to listen to Dire Straits when I do her. When you "dance," you just listen to the music and stroke with the beat or a variation on the beat. There is no choreography for this dance. Keep communicating and remember to use short strokes, as many doers' strokes tend to become too long. Both men and woman can have fun checking out different types of music and seeing which best suit their orgasms.

## Power Games

Although being playful is fun, sometimes men have to be serious to get a woman's attention. Power games—including coercion, fear, and pain—are methods that you can use to get your partner to feel more. However, you must communicate before using any of these techniques. Before you slap, pinch, or cause pain to someone, you *must* get their permission. You also have to know what you are doing, and when you slap or pinch, you must do it at the right time and stay in constant communication. Some people have issues around this area, and you must refrain from using any of these techniques on them.

Power games aren't the first techniques to use either, but they're good to include in your bag of tricks, and you can use them when they are appropriate.

Coercion is a way to get your partner to feel more. It's somewhat similar to seduction: When she doesn't come toward you, it's best to push her away. Although she is able to come really well, she may demonstrate some resistance and hold out in some area. If you've done her before and know that she can get off on the first stroke, but when you touch her this time there's little or no sensation, don't keep rubbing and don't hope that she'll start feeling more. It's time to communicate what you feel.

Tell her—in a nice, friendly way at first, telling the truth without anger—that perhaps she really doesn't want to enjoy pleasure at this time. Your next step depends on her reaction. If she agrees with you, that is a good sign that she may want to go for more pleasure. If she argues, that is a sure sign that more extreme measures have to be taken. It would be wise at this point to tell her to put on her clothes, and then talk to each other. It is okay to be tougher with an experienced person than with someone who has little experience. You can tell her how you love doing her, that you notice she isn't feeling much, and that maybe it would be best to do something else. She will respect you for telling her the truth, and even if she does not take up your offer this time, she may the next time.

If you find yourself working too hard at doing her, let her know that you want her coming to be easy and tell her that if you have to work this hard, you will stop rubbing. It is best to make sure that you don't come off sounding like a mean and vindictive person. This can be done by making sure that you are not acting out of anger, but as a friend whose main interest is your partner's genuine pleasure.

Why do women sometimes resist? Many women have a fear of orgasm. They believe that if they surrender to you, they will lose their functioning and reasoning abilities. They will become your slave and have no mind of their own. People don't like to owe others. Women also know that many men function from a "now that I've rubbed your back, you can rub mine" philosophy.

You have to make it clear to her that you are doing her for your own pleasure and she owes you nothing in return. If you tell her the truth in a nice way and maybe use a bit of coercion for seduction, you will find that she will trust you more and that her fear of orgasm may be replaced by her fear that you will stop.

Fear and pain are other ways to get her attention. By slapping her pussy or her buttocks or tugging on her pubic hair slightly more than she expected, you can overcome her fear of orgasm. If she says that she isn't feeling anything, using more pressure, such as slapping or tugging or pinching, can be tried (remember to ask permission first). Then ask her if she can feel that. The goal is not to hurt her, but to get her into her body and into feeling sensation. Sometimes just the thought of being slapped can make her feel her genitals more and erotically stimulate her. Women can also use different pressures and slaps when playing with a man's genitals.

In addition to slapping or "spanking" other erogenous areas, you can spank the clitoris, the most sensitive place. This should only be done with total agreement. You can slap with two or more fingers. With a short snap of the wrist, the fingers sting the clitoris. Again, find out which pressures she prefers. We hardly ever use slapping in our sex acts. When we have, it has only been one slap on the clitoris, and then we immediately bring the woman up for a peak with regular stroking. Not all women like to be slapped, so this is not for everyone.

Some people like to be slapped with a whip. Whips can be purchased at adult sex stores. If you do get into whipping, it is a good idea to create a special code word to let your partner know when you really have had enough. However, we do not wish to go into more detail about S&M here, because we use slapping to get a partner's attention and to get them to feel their body more. Although slapping and whipping can be fun, it's best not to depend on them to replace or initiate orgasm every time. These are erotic techniques and, as we've said elsewhere, eroticism can be a spice but not the main meal.

# ⤳ Fantasy ⤳

Everyone's mind holds viewpoints and thoughts. Almost everyone has an imagination. Everyone, supposedly, has a dream life, both night dreams and daydreams. We all also have fantasies, both sexual and otherwise. This ability to create conceptual thoughts is our sixth sense.

Many things can add to a sensual experience, and we believe that all of them are fine as long as they do no one any harm. Such additions include things that please our five senses: adding beautiful music, wonderful smells, fabulous tastes, sensational touches, and gorgeous sights. They can also include things that please our sixth sense, such as fantasies that turn on you or your partner.

Our bodies cannot tell the difference between real and imagined thoughts. If we think that there is a burglar in the basement, our bodies respond with the same adrenaline rush that they do if there actually is a prowler in our basement—even if it's only the wind making some noise. We have a friend whose father was not allowed to watch football games because he got too excited and his heart could not take the excitement. He was not playing in the game, but his body responded as if he was involved. Sexual fantasies can work in the same way, stimulating a dull sex life or making a good one much more exciting.

The only possible danger is that we might get off only on the fantasy and on nothing else. Then the fantasy becomes a perversion, which means that it develops an exclusive nature. Only being able to get off in the missionary position in the dark with the man on top would be considered a perversion. But most people, fortunately, can get off in a myriad of ways, and adding fantasy to the mix only makes for more fun. Our imagination is extremely powerful. It can add a lot of spice and fun to our lives if we let it.

Men and women generally fantasize differently. This is not a fact etched in stone, but in our experience, men have shorter, less-intricate fantasies. They usually involve specific sensual acts that he has done or could imagine doing with people he knows or has seen. Their fantasies usually are quite visual and may leap from frame to frame like an old-fashioned Rolodex or a flickering computer screen. They may consist of only female body parts, such as thighs, pussies, or breasts. He might fantasize that he's dominated sexually: His girlfriend, scantily dressed and wearing high heels, ties him to a bed and has her way with him. Alternately, he might do the dominating and have his way with a woman. We've had more than one student who fantasized about watching his girlfriend with another man. We have known men who fantasized about having sex with many women at once.

We also have known women who fantasized about having sex with many men, having all their orifices filled at once. We've had female students who fantasized about dominating men sexually or about being dominated or even raped. The biggest difference between women's and men's fantasies is that women's fantasies are more involved. That is why men like to look at girlie magazines and women prefer romance novels. Women's fantasies often have lots of dialogue and costumes and more of a plot. They might get to a sexual act only at the end of their fantasies, if at all. Women's fantasies often are about people they haven't met, like Robert Redford or Brad Pitt, or some wild animal; men, on the other hand, usually fantasize about someone they know, knew in the past, or saw that day. Some men, of course, also fantasize about celebrities, such as Pamela Anderson Lee or Christie Brinkley. We've met women who have short visual fantasies and men who have longer fantasies than the average male.

All these fantasies are wonderful, and there obviously is no right fantasy. You can be as naughty and far out as you like. As long as it adds to your experience, go for it. When I masturbate, I almost always fantasize. Some people don't fantasize as much; any amount is okay. As long as you are not hurting anyone or allowing your fantasy to become exclusive, it's fine to fantasize about whatever you like. It's okay to fantasize about animals or homosexual acts if they turn you on. There's no law against fantasizing, and any restrictions that anyone dictates only stifle our creative abilities.

You can share your fantasies with your partner and play with only those that you want to use. For example, when you're doing your partner, you can tell them one of their favorite fantasies, using it to enhance the experience. Some people like to act out their fantasies, but others want to keep them just as fantasies. You can talk about this with your partner and find out whether they want you to playact their fantasies with them.

We knew a man who had a fantasy about being tied up and whipped by his girlfriend. She was reluctant to do it, but finally, on his birthday, she decided to give him that gift and play the dominatrix role. She dressed up in high heels and a special outfit. She had a lot of fun preparing for and doing it, and they both enjoyed the experience. It is not something that they want to do every time they have sex, but the memory of that experience is a fantasy that they can use again and again.

When having sex with your partner, you can add fun to the experience by talking about your fantasy about someone or something else, unless your partner has difficulty with that. The fantasy doesn't mean you actually want to be with that other person, and your partner probably will be turned on by the idea and your honesty. You will also feel better, as you won't have to feel guilty or sneaky about the fantasy once you've expressed yourself. Some people may have problems if you talk about someone else during sex, and in that case it's probably best not to bring it up.

We knew a couple who were considered quite open sexually. Her husband could talk about almost any fantasy that he had, except for fantasies about one woman whom she did not like and of whom she was jealous. He learned the hard way: His wife threw a fit when he brought the name of that other woman to bed. He did not repeat that mistake.

Fantasy is something to add to the experience. It is a form of eroticism and can spice up an experience, but it is not the "main meal" that will sustain you, and you will get into trouble if you rely on fantasy to have a good time. You do not have to add fantasy to have a good sex life, but its addition can make your sex life even better.

## Begging

Sometimes, when you do someone, they say that they want you to continue touching them, but you feel they've had enough. In these moments, trust yourself. This is a great time to communicate what is going on, and it even opens up an opportunity for your partner to beg you to rub them. Begging can be a fun game to play, and it can add to the experience. We've known couples who have had a lot of fun with it.

Begging usually consists of being extremely polite, rather than actually groveling. Some of the lines we have heard include: "Will you please rub me some more, kind sir (kind madam)?" and "Please, don't stop." It is a way to get your partner to admit that they are being pleasured, and it allows them to express their surrender. Remember that the surrender is to their own greater pleasure, not to some superior person. Some people really get into role-playing, assuming dominant or submissive (top or bottom) roles. This is fine as long as it's played between consenting adults and they properly communicate with each other. We are not experts in this area, however, so we advise you to find appropriate books or groups to learn more.

Of course, if your partner's begging doesn't feel sincere, let them know. If you or your partner feel that the begging game is sexist or morally wrong, you are not required to play it in order to experience a great orgasm.

## Advanced Doing

A number of women are able to have great orgasms. Most of them have trained their bodies to be able to experience a great deal of pleasure. The amount of training that's needed depends on the woman. We have met some women who, almost immediately after finding out that EMOs were available, were able to experience them, so they needed very little training. But most people need more time to train their bodies to feel that much pleasure. We use the term "advanced doing" to describe doing someone who can already have long, intense orgasms.

Women who, like Vera, have trained their bodies to feel a lot of pleasure are able to get off even before you touch them. They can come if you blow air on their genitals or through heavy pressure. They can orgasm and have strong contractions if they're touched anywhere around the vicinity of their clitorises.

They can tell immediately if you are on their spot, but they can get off very well even if you're not. They have even bigger and more intense orgasms if you're on the spot and know when to peak them. These advanced comers are a lot of fun, and they're easy to do. They can talk easily about what they feel and are able to report all specific experiences of pleasure while they're being done. They can tell you what they like while you do them, and they can help you succeed.

Of course, you still have to pay attention to what you are doing and remember when to take breaks and when to peak your partner. Advanced doing is the same as the doing that we've written about elsewhere in this book. The basic requirements are identical: You keep your attention on your partner and notice where she is. You go with your feelings. However, with an advanced "doee," the breaks are usually shorter, the peaks are longer, and she's ready to go for more pleasure in a split second.

Sometimes, women who can get off really well become lazy at it. If this happens, you must point it out in a friendly way at first. Usually, once you catch her being lazy or not coming as well as she could, she's grateful that you noticed and will get off like a bandit in the future. After all, if you, the doer, have been lazy and let her get away with mediocre orgasms, you cannot expect her to respond to your touch with her greatest orgasm in the future either. Of course, having mediocre orgasms sometimes is okay—just remember to point it out and to notice what's going on.

Intention is a very important skill when doing an advanced "doee." Intention can be described as using your focus and attention to produce an effect in the universe. In this case, you intend to bring another person's energy level higher or lower, depending on what you feel in your own body. By having strong intention, you can bring people up with almost any stroke and can also bring them down with the same stroke. The only difference is your intention. A good way to demonstrate intention is through direct, spoken instructions, which are very effective on sexually trained women.

With your full attention and intention, the advanced "doee" will be able to have—at worst—a wonderful time and a great orgasm. At best, she might just have the best orgasm of her life.

## ✐ Coming Together ✐

Before you can come together, you and your partner must be good at doing. The **coming together position** is one in which you do each other at the same time. Before we describe it, however, remember that communication is of the utmost importance when coming together. If communication lags, the "Coming Demons" will torment you. But you can exorcise them with precise and pertinent communication, and when they're gone, coming together becomes one of the most ecstatic experiences you can have.

The coming together position is especially useful for women, who are often curious about the most pleasurable way to deal with a man's genitals. The most pleasurable way to deal with anything—including genitals—is via orgasm. This position gives her the opportunity to do just that.

The woman lies on her back. The man lies on his side (on his right side if left-handed, on his left side if right-handed) facing the opposite direction. His head is near his partner's genitals, and his partner's head is near his genitals. This way, his hands can touch his partner's genitals and he can see them as well. They should use lots of pillows to prop themselves up and to help them stay in a relaxed, comfortable position. Place large pillows behind you, for support, and rest your arm upon a smaller pillow.

It's best to start by stroking the woman first. The man lies on his left side with his left arm (if he's right-handed) between her legs, resting on his forearm. She lies on her back. His upper torso, meanwhile, rests comfortably upon a pillow that is on her left thigh. He can then use his right hand to stroke her genitals, just as we described in the regular doing positions. He can tease, lubricate her genitals, and start stroking with lots of communication, letting her know what he is doing at all times. Once she is receiving regular, repeated, pleasurable strokes and is coming easily, he can pretty much lie back while continuing to stroke. She can then rise onto her side and begin to pleasure her partner while he pleasures her. Using some lubricant that's been placed conveniently nearby, she can play with his cock.

If she so desires, she can place the head of his penis in her mouth, keeping her lips soft and her mouth above the crown of his penis, as she continues to stroke with her hands. She shouldn't bob her head up and down but should use her mouth to feel and give pleasure. And remember that communication needs to be ongoing—it is difficult to talk with a cock in your mouth, so this part is really recommended for advanced students. And the male partner needs to do lots of talking if she has her mouth occupied.

Competition for attention and selfishness are what cause "Coming Demons" to thrive. If you're thinking that your partner should put more attention on your genitals, or if you're wondering whether to feel your genitals or put more attention on your partner's, you are in your head rather than feeling. This is the time to communicate and even take a break if necessary. You want to continuously have and give attention, not feel that you need attention. You can tame the "Coming Demons" if you enthusiastically enjoy yourself, do what feels best, and communicate. You use the same techniques as in ordinary doing: use peaking, take breaks, and do lots of talking.

When you do this position properly, energy circulates through your bodies in a way that's analogous to a cyclotron's energy. The more you approve of and appreciate what is happening, the higher you're able to go. Before you start this exercise, you can decide how long you wish to continue it. Remember that you are touching for your own pleasure, not for any effect.

Here's an example of coming together. A man and woman decide to use the standard coming together position. They talk about how they will lie on the bed, and they gather all the necessary pillows. The man wants a couple of large pillows to place behind him to support his back. He wants a medium-size pillow to place on the woman's thigh and a small pillow to place under his doing arm. The woman wants a pillow to place under her outside thigh, a large pillow near at hand that she can use to support her back when she moves onto her side, and a pillow to place under her head. They each have some Vaseline and a washcloth nearby. They agree to do this position for twenty-five minutes and at that point to decide if they want to continue or do something else. They set the alarm clock for twenty-five minutes.

At first, the woman lies on her back. The man lies on his left side, stuffing the large pillow behind his back. He places his left hand under the woman's buttocks, resting his forearm between her legs. He rests his side upon a pillow placed over her thigh. His right arm is free to reach for lubricant, and he can rest his right elbow on a small pillow on her abdomen.

After teasing her pubic hair and different parts of her pussy, he lets her know that he is going to put some lubricant on her clitoris. He puts some lubricant on her perineum and on her inner lips, and then he puts some lubricant directly on her clitoris and starts to take her up. She really enjoys his strokes and acknowledges all the wonderful sensations that she experiences. He reports all signs of orgasm and tells her how wonderful her genitals feel and smell. He peaks her by skipping a stroke and then starts taking her up again. He takes her for a couple more peaks, and she really gets off well.

She puts some lubricant on her hands. As she moves from her back to her side, getting comfortable with the proper pillow arrangement, she informs him that she will put the lubrication on him. He keeps stroking and lets her know how exquisite her hands on his cock feel. She tells him that she is going to hold his cock before stroking it. She tells him how engorged he is becoming and how great her pussy feels. They now go up together, both stroking, for a great peak, acknowledging the whole time. They stop at about the same time, tell each other how much fun they are having, and agree to start stroking again. They peak together a number of times, going higher with each peak.

He lies on his back now, still stroking her clitoris. Her orgasm is taking him higher, and his is taking her higher at the same time. She tells him that she is going to ejaculate him on the next peak and that there is nothing that he can do to stop her. She takes him higher and higher, feeling her pussy at the same time. He gets a secondary erection, his cock purple and bulbous, as he starts ejaculating in her hands, and then she lightens and slows down her stroke, extending the orgasm. After lying in sheer ecstasy for a while, he gets back onto his side and gives her a pull-up as she continues to have strong contractions. They towel each other off just as the alarm rings.

You can come together in variations of the position described above. One position that we sometimes use is the **bonobo position.** The man sits over the woman in the ordinary doing position. After she has started to get off well, she puts some lubricant on his cock and strokes it with her hand or against her thigh without having to move her body. Both people can orgasm pleasurably together. Of course, communication still needs to be top-notch in this position.

By this point in the book, you have come a long way. You've learned about basic and advanced EMO techniques and the skills and communication that are necessary to have and produce this pleasure. But, like the old proverb says, "Everything that goes up must come down." It is now time to come down, and in the rest of the book we provide a lot of information about human sexuality and sexual health that will help to bring you down. Coming down is not bad; it is just a different direction from up. If you wish to go higher again, you can always go back and reread the previous pages later and maybe even read them out loud with your partner, if you have not done so already. But now it is time to enjoy the descent.

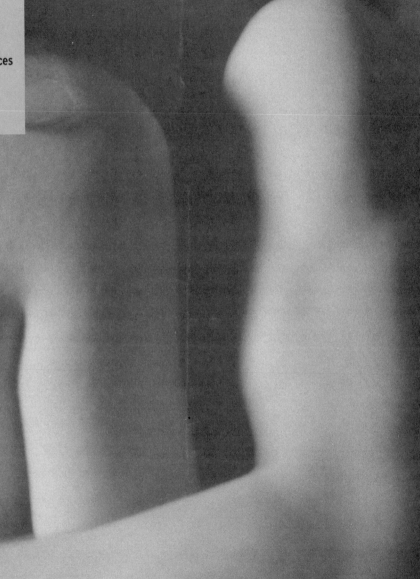

*Coming Down*

# CHAPTER 10

# Heat Cycles

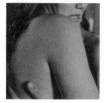

*I*n his book *The Last Panda,* the zoologist George B. Schaller explains the heat cycle of these bears, which live in the hills of China. They basically eat only bamboo, chomping on the leaves, stems, or shoots, depending upon what time of the year it is. There is not much nutrition in bamboo, so they have to eat a large quantity to stay alive. They do not have time to do much more than eat and sleep. They can't even hibernate, because bamboo doesn't put enough weight on them. They are solitary animals and do not live as couples or in a group. Each panda keeps to its own territory, which is fairly big, as they have to graze on large quantities of bamboo.

Female pandas go into heat only about once a year. At this time, a male may leave his own territory for that of the receptive female. When he gets there, he may find other males already there. The males might fight, or a least try to scare one another off, so they can get a chance to mate with the female. She is receptive for a number of days, during which time more than one male may get to mount her. She might reject some of the suitors. After mating (or getting beaten up or rejected), the males head back to their individual territories. The female is no longer in heat and won't be for another year. If she has been impregnated, she'll be out of circulation for at least two years.[19]

Many people assume that humans, unlike pandas, don't have heat cycles. Yet in fact, heat cycles are common to all mammals. Although we sometimes pretend to be above nature, human beings are mammals and are affected by the seasons and natural bodily cycles.

This chapter includes information on many kinds of human heat cycles, including the menstrual cycle and the annual heat cycle. We also discuss two kinds of heat that don't occur in cycles: situational and volitional heat, which can happen at any time. Volitional heat, as demonstrated by female human beings, is the most important type of all. She can decide to have sex whenever and wherever she pleases; she need not wait for any special time or place. Her volitional heat trumps all other forms of heat, including the menstrual cycle. The chapter concludes with an explanation of why women developed volitional heat and explores how we humans compare to our closest ancestors, especially the bonobo apes.

## The Menstrual Cycle

In most girls, menses start between the ages of ten and thirteen. Recent research indicates that the age of menarche (the onset of menses) may be dropping due to something in the environment, although scientists are unsure what that factor may be. Stress can also cause early menarche. Some women whom we know started menstruating quite early due to stress; one woman, who was imprisoned in a Nazi concentration camp at age nine, subsequently experienced very early menarche.

This rite of passage is sometimes celebrated for the gift of life that it promises but is sometimes also derided as "the curse," as our society usually calls it. One woman friend got her period when she was ten. She was very disturbed because she did not know what was happening to her. She took a cold bath, which stopped the bleeding, but it began again once she was out of the tub. She bathed a number of times before she asked her mother what was happening. This incident occurred a number of years ago, but many young girls still go through trauma at menarche. If parents felt more comfortable and could tell girls about their menstrual cycle before it began, describing it in a positive way, girls would not have to experience such confusion.

The menstrual cycle runs for about twenty-eight to thirty-two days and then repeats itself. Most women experience two different peaks of sexual receptivity, or heat, every month. One of the peaks is ovulation, which is accompanied by an increase in estrogen. A woman is most responsive to having intercourse at this time. Many women report a feeling of well-being and clear thinking during ovulation. The window for creating a baby is very small, probably less than seventy-two hours. It isn't always easy to determine when ovulation occurs and thus when a woman is in heat. (Other mammals give clearer signs.) A temperature test can help determine when she is most receptive, but the exact time is still difficult to discern.

Many women experience a second peak during the days just before their menses. Although estrogen levels are down at this point, progesterone levels also fall, which leaves more "binding sites" (hormonal receptor sites on cells) available for testosterone. Testosterone is the male sex hormone, but women also have it, albeit in lower amounts than men. This second heat is easier to detect because a woman experiences some bloating before her period. She may have a musky odor. Her pupils tend to be more dilated. She may have a "pregnancy mask" (a trace of extra skin pigment) under her eyes. She may crave gooey or salty, fatty foods, such as chocolate or potato chips. She may be irritable. In fact, a name (pre-menstrual syndrome, or PMS) has been coined to describe this time period.

Although a woman may not desire intercourse during this time, it's a great time to relieve her pressure and use it for pleasure. (It's also among the safer times for intercourse, as pregnancy is somewhat less likely.) The best way to relieve her pressure is an intense orgasm, and the best, most efficient way to give her such an orgasm is to take control of the nervous system via "doing." Her excess energy during this time is the fuel for a great orgasm. The added engorgement at this time can be thought of as potential orgasm instead of potential pain. Many women have their most intense orgasms at this time. However, a man must be at his seductive best to convince a woman to get done during this period because, as we've noted, among the signs of PMS is irritability. We've known many women who suffered severe cramps before their periods, but with lots of genital attention, especially of the EMO kind, their cramps wondrously disappeared.

Physical activities apart from sex can also help to detumesce a woman in heat—they're just not as pleasurable. Physical exercise such as running, aerobics, and weight-lifting can bring her down. So, too, can cleaning, scrubbing, or polishing around the house. Massage is also detumescing, especially deep-tissue massage. Any kind of attention from a lover or a friend, especially listening to her, produces some relief.

If you do a woman during this period, it's a good idea to spend extra time bringing her down with firm pressure and attention. Also, remember that there is a good possibility that a few hours after a woman has come down from this sexual pressure, she'll be back up there again and will require further detumescing.

After the first couple of days of menstrual bleeding, this intense pressure has receded. The days after her period and the few days after her ovulation are the times of the month when she is at her lowest heat. Of course, she can still have great sex and great orgasms during these times.

## ✎ Annual Heat Cycle ✎

Human beings are mammals, named after the mammary glands (breasts). We are warm-blooded animals that respond to fluctuations in our environment, including changes in temperature, humidity, and other climatic variables. We try to modify our environment by the use of heating in winter and air-conditioning in summer, in both our homes and vehicles. In spite of our modified environment, however, we are still affected by seasonal changes. We call this response to the cycle of seasonal change the annual heat cycle.

Like the menstrual cycle, the annual heat cycle has two high points and two low points. The high points are spring and fall, and the low points are winter and summer. Whether this is due to temperature, the angle of the sun's rays, or both is not known, but this cycle has been well demonstrated in agrarian societies. The busiest time of year, the time when the most energy is available, is spring, when farmers get the soil ready and plant their crops. The second-highest energy level occurs in fall, when harvesting is done. During the two low periods, winter and summer, agrarian societies don't need as much energy, as people sharpen their tools in winter and water, weed, and watch their crops grow in summer.

Winter, especially late December and January in the Northern Hemisphere, is the time of year with the lowest energy. Many animals are hibernating or just trying to survive. When spring comes, the ice melts and animals start to appear from their burrows. This is the time of year when many animals mate.

Although we don't hibernate, we're also at our lowest energy level in the winter months, and with the onset of spring our energy level takes a big jump. Human beings find the energy to do spring cleaning, start wars, and create riots. We're affected by the renewed natural activity around us. We even say that some people who are especially affected by this energy have "spring fever." Once the hot days of summer roll around, we have much less energy for either sex or fighting, especially during the "dog days" of July and August. Once the weather cools off again, our energy increases as children return to school and grown-ups return to work. By Christmas and the New Year, the energy has settled down again. Perhaps this is why it's difficult to get up the energy to have fun at a New Year's party!

The cycle repeats itself year after year. In the Southern Hemisphere, the cycles are reversed, yet spring and fall are still the two high points. Even in

California, which has year-round nice weather, we have the same heat cycles, and spring and fall bring forth an abundance of energy.

## ✒ Situational Heat ✒

Male mammals don't experience estrus or go into heat, yet they do seem to affect the female population. In many primates that live in groups, a new male entering the group causes the females to go into heat. He gets a lot of attention when he's new.

Similarly, when we have been involved in communal situations among people, we've noticed that when a new male member enters the group, many women are attracted to him and check him out. They may try him out sexually, and he may believe himself to be a stud. After a few months, however, the women all lose interest in him, or perhaps one woman takes him on in a more permanent way. When he first arrives, he thinks he's died and gone to heaven. Then reality returns, the women leave him alone, and he wonders what he's done wrong.

Women who live together or even spend lots of time together tend to go into heat together. We knew a group of women who lived in the same house; they were quite close to one another and spent a lot of time together. They all had their periods at the same time. When a new woman joined the group, her cycle changed to become synchronous with the rest. A number of scientific studies have been done on this phenomenon, and researchers have come up with different results. It seems to depend on what kind of relationship the women have with one another. If they do not get along, they do not influence one another's cycles, or they may even influence their friends to menstruate at different times. It's also been reported that women who spend time around men have more regular menstrual cycles than women who do not. There may be a substance in male sweat that produces this effect. In these studies, women's menstrual cycles have been shown to go from unpredictable to predictable within a short period of time after they were exposed to male sweat.

## Volitional Heat

Unlike most mammals, human females can have sex whenever they decide to. They don't have to be ovulating or premenstrual, and it doesn't have to be springtime. Women just have to desire it. Human males don't really have this option. Their vote is almost always "yes," but their desire has no specific "heat" effect on the women in their lives. If a man initiates sex by forcing himself on a woman, that is called rape. But that doesn't mean he can't flirt and seduce a woman into desiring him.

A man may not be attracted to a woman, but if she turns up her heat high enough, he soon will be. This is a gift from our female ancestors, who probably traded sex for goods and services in order to survive long enough to pass us their genes.

Volitional heat enables a woman to desire sex for whatever reason she likes. There's nothing on TV, she's not hungry, and she doesn't feel like reading. She can decide to go for sensual pleasure instead. Doing is a perfect answer to volitional heat, because any time is a great time for doing or getting done. She doesn't have to worry about getting pregnant or a disease. She does not have to feel any special heat, in fact. She just has to be turned on to wanting pleasure for herself. If she admits to feeling flat when she feels flat, she can start to get pleasure from that point. Not admitting it makes it difficult for her to go up. Appreciation, approval, curiosity, and turn-on will all increase her heat. We've gone for many a fine ride after we admitted that we felt flat.

## Menopause

All women encounter menopause, and it can be the best time of their lives, sensually and otherwise. Human females, unlike most animals, live thirty to fifty years after their fertile period has ended. Around the age of fifty, women undergo another huge hormonal shift. Their ovaries become nonfunctional and no longer produce follicles or the resultant eggs. Women no longer have a menstrual period: hence the name *menopause*.

According to the scientist Kristen Hawkes, Natalie Angier writes in *Woman: An Intimate Geography,* women evolved this ability to live past fertility because of their usefulness to younger members of their groups. Groups with older female members survived better than those without such members, so these groups tended to propagate genes for longevity. Because genes are not sexually biased and male children receive more than half their genes from their mothers, longevity genes are inherited by male babies as well, whose lives have also been extended. This theory was originally introduced in the 1950s as the "Grandmother Hypothesis." It fell out of favor, but some scientists have revived it.

Our society is very difficult for older women, as we are youth worshippers. Society values a woman according to her attractiveness and thus doesn't often value older women. Men aren't so concerned with their appearance, as they are judged upon their productivity more than their looks. Thus, menopause is a very difficult time for women. Many of Vera's relatives went crazy at this time; a few even killed themselves. Vera did not know what to expect when she went through menopause. During this time, she decided to have a lot of attention put on her orgasm and on pleasure. She decided to have long orgasms daily. She breezed through menopause without a problem. She is almost fifteen years past menopause now, and she recommends orgasm to anyone who wants to pleasurably experience it. One person does not make an experiment, of course, and we have no proof that everyone who orgasms regularly has an easy time with menopause. We do feel that regular intense orgasms make menopause more enjoyable, if not easier.

During menopause, estrogen levels fall because the ovaries no longer function. Other cells and tissues still produce some estrogen, however. The loss of estrogen seems to have no effect on the clitoris's function, response, or ability to experience pleasure. Nonetheless, many women start hormone replacement therapy after menopause for a variety of reasons. Vera did not take any hormone replacements, but that is a personal choice that each person must make, and it does not mean that she won't take any in the future. If you are entering menopause, it is a good idea to read up on hormone replacement therapy. It has many pros and cons, and recent improvements in medicine mean that a wide choice of hormones is available and individuals can choose the ones that work best for them. Some women may choose to take hormones right away; others, like Vera, may wait to take them or never take them at all.[20]

Many women give up sex altogether when they get older, but this does not have to be the case. You do not need functioning ovaries to experience great orgasms. We know a number of postmenopausal women whose orgasms keep getting better. Their children are finally out of the house, and they have more time to enjoy themselves. Menopause can be a great time to put attention on your body and experience more pleasure than ever before. The more positive attention that you put on yourself and the more you learn to like yourself the way you are, the more sex appeal you'll have and the more attractive others will find you.

## Sex Dealers

In this section, we will explore humans' divergence from our primate ancestors, particularly in our ability to have sex at will. We will also explore some anthropological similarities and differences between ourselves and other primates and will explain why ovulation is hidden in humans. We have included this information to help you better understand volitional heat and how and why it developed in humans. We believe the better we understand our closest relatives and their sexual similarities and differences from us, the better we will be able to know our place in nature and our capacity for pleasure.

According to Helen Fisher's *The Sex Contract*, female humans developed their ability to have sex at will once we came out of the trees and learned to walk on two legs instead of the four legs employed by other primates. When a female in heat stands up on two legs, her heat is less obvious because her genitals are more hidden than they would be if she stood on all fours. At the same time, the heads of newborns became larger because our brains and brain capacity continued to evolve.[21]

As newborns' head sizes increased and women's pelvic frames narrowed in order to accommodate their new erect posture, births began to occur earlier in gestation. As a result, babies were more immature at birth. Tending these babies meant that women could no longer hunt or gather food as effectively as they had in the past—it is difficult to carry an infant around on two legs, and the newborns could no longer clutch their mothers' backs in the way that primate young do. Thus women stayed close to camp.

Fisher argues that our ancient female ancestors benefited by getting another person to help feed them and their children. They traded sex for food, assistance, and protection. To gain the best and most protein for themselves and their children, women who could have the most sex survived and were the most fit to reproduce again. Their children also survived and were the most fit to reproduce. This survival of the fittest, over an extended time, selected sexual "athletes" who, like modern women, could have sex without being in heat. The women who survived were those who could have sex at any time, even when pregnant or weaning a child, just because they wanted to. Fisher's idea is, of course, only a theory, and it may never be proved. In fact, some anthropologists believe that in many early hunting and gathering societies, the amount of meat that hunters brought back was actually very limited, so women wouldn't have had much incentive to use sex in return for food. Even so, an alignment with a man or a number of men would have been beneficial for the safety of a woman and her infant.

In our studies, we've found that young women under thirty (or sometimes a bit older than thirty) are more like "dealers" or "pushers" of sex than actual users of sex. This means that they don't have sex for themselves because of the pleasure it brings them, but do it in exchange for goods and services from their lovers or for emotional rewards, such as love or a feeling of security. The dating game simulates the food-for-sex scenario that may have evolved among our ancestors—this may be why men usually pay for dinner, thinking that if they spend enough money, they'll be rewarded with sex. We've known women who were exceptions to this rule, of course, women who could, in their twenties, go for pleasure for pleasure's sake and learn to have EMOs.

Of course, the food-for-sex game has become a bit outdated for modern women and men. Modern women aren't totally dependent on men or on another person to rear a child. There are more single women successfully raising children alone than ever before (although they usually still receive help from their mothers or friends). One friend of ours deliberately conceived without telling the man; she's raised the child alone to be a fine young man, but she's gotten help from her mother and other relatives. Only in the last twenty-five years of the twentieth century have women deliberately chosen to raise children without a father. Before that point, raising a child as a single mother was usually done by default when women were widowed or abandoned by their husbands. There are also some families in which the father is the sole parent, but this is usually because the mother has died or left.

Men cannot tell when women can be impregnated. There are no major physical signs, as there are in other animals. Why is women's ovulation hidden from them as well as from men? This question is still being debated by scientists. Most female animals can accept penile insertion only during estrus, the period during when they can become pregnant. Hormones cause the females to go into heat, and they become receptive to and noticed by the males. Most primates, including the apes and monkeys (our closest relatives), experience obvious estrus (many female primates show engorged and reddened genitals that are visible to the males). Female primates' bodies can accept penile insertion throughout their cycle, but they're only interested in it when they're in noticeable heat.

Since men cannot be sure that the woman is in estrus and can become pregnant, they do not know for sure that the offspring produced is theirs. They also don't know for sure that their offspring is *not* theirs. Paternity is a more important issue for humans than it is for other primates, as human fathers usually participate much more than other male animals do in raising offspring. Many male animals just deposit their semen; that's the end of their job. Human fathers generally assist in the feeding and teaching of children. With so much time and effort at stake, men don't want to raise another man's offspring. (We're speaking from the perspective of our genes—we don't mean to imply that some men don't want to be stepfathers or adopt children.) Humans lived as hunter-gatherers for most of our history. In a hunter-gatherer society, it wasn't uncommon for more than one male to help a woman raise a child. A man knew that he could be the father of the child, and so he wanted to help rear the child, even if the woman had more than one lover. This uncertainty also usually prevented men from killing a mother's children out of jealousy, because the children might have been their own.

## ✎ Bonobos and Other ✎ Monkey Business

The ability to have volitional sex may be in our genes. Humans and the bonobo (or pygmy) chimpanzee—our closest relative, along with the common chimpanzee, on the evolutionary tree—are the only apes known to have volitional sex. All three types of primate shared a common ancestor approximately eight million years ago. Humans also share 98.3 percent of the other primates' genes.

As we've said earlier in this book, we believe that turn-on is the natural state. By considering bonobo apes, we can see the possibility of living with more turn-on and the possibility of a society in which female pleasure comes first. Bonobos have sex even more often than humans, for any reason whatsoever. Sex is a way of life for the bonobos: It is the first method that they use to settle disputes and make decisions about matters such as who gets to eat first. They engage in female-female as well as male-female sex. They have genital-genital, oral-genital, and hand-genital contact. Bonobos have been seen kissing each other on the lips, performing oral sex, and even engaging in a sort of French kissing. They have very large clitorises (humans don't have the largest ones in the primate world), which are clearly visible. When they're in heat, they don't hide the fact.

Unlike the other primates, where the larger males have first dibs on the food, the female bonobos get first choice. The females lead the group, and if a male is causing trouble, the females conspire together and gang up on him.[22] Like humans, bonobos can walk upright (as well as on all fours).

Some primates, such as gorillas, live in groups where one male does most of the mating with the females in his harem. He mates with them only when they're in heat. Other primates, such as the common chimpanzee, live in groups that have a hierarchy of males and females, but in these groups more than one male gets to mate with the females. Again, however, they mate only when the females are in heat. Some primates form pair bonds similar to those between humans, but they're less adulterous than we are. One such animal is the gibbon, which lives in isolated pair bonds. Kim Wallen, Natalie Angier writes in *Woman: An Intimate Geography*, has reported that rhesus monkeys will have sex with a member of their group even if the female's not in heat, but the monkey couples do this only when they're alone. If other members of the group are around, sex does not happen unless the female is in heat.[23]

The size of primates' testes varies according to the ways that the primate has evolved. Chimpanzees, which are smaller than humans, have larger genitals than we do because there is a lot of competition for mating. To ensure that the young are fathered by them rather than by another chimpanzee, males need a lot of sperm; thus they have large testes. Although male gorillas are larger than men, their genitals are a lot smaller than ours. There is very little sexual competition among male gorillas once a male has risen to lead a harem and become the "alpha male," so only a small amount of sperm is needed to ensure reproduction. The alpha male is still challenged by other males who physically try to dethrone him, but females will usually only mate with the reigning champion. Human males have moderate to large testes compared to those of other primates. This is probably due to the fact that though there usually is pair bonding, humans do stray and have affairs, and thus fatherhood could be questionable.[24]

In this chapter, we have described how humans are similar to other mammals, especially the primates, and how our own evolution has created differences. Although we share many characteristics and genes with our primate relatives, we are the only primate whose brain has developed a huge frontal lobe. We are the only animal that has been able to create great science and great art and pass our achievements on to others through books, teaching, and now the computer. We're also the only animal that has learned how to produce EMOs. None of the other primates, including the bonobo, has been able to learn how to produce EMOs, but then again, no human culture other than our own has been able to learn how to do it either.

# CHAPTER 11

# Conscious Choices

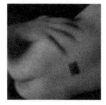

**M**any people are victims of their upbringing and their emotions. They do not realize that they have the choice to create their lives and shape them to be the way that they want. In this chapter, we'll demonstrate how people keep repeating losing behavior and explain what they can do to start winning, which is enormously helpful when you're learning how to experience and create EMOs. We will also describe some options that people can use to turn themselves from victims into winners.

# The White Knight

There was a maiden, a lovely sight,
Waiting lonely for her knight in white.
She checked out all available men,
But they never made a salable ten.
The miller too fat, the butcher too bloody.
Some were too pale, some were too ruddy.
Some were too poor or too fuddy-duddy.
Daily she waited upon her front porch,
Still praying that she'd be passed the torch.
Out in the distance, a cloud of dust.
A gentle stirring in her bust.
Closer the shape began to form.
Could this be the end to her lonely storm?
A knight it was, as white as can be,
Upon a steed, riding most nobly.
He stopped at her door and got off his horse.
He said he was there to aid her course.
She said, "That's great; now let me see.
Would you kill a dragon for me?"
"That's my duty," the knight replied,
Being a veteran of dragoncide.
Off he went, back onto his horse,
Straight off to kill without remorse.
He cut off the dragon's ears and the tail,
And returned to the maiden without fail.
She said, "That's great; now let me see.
Would you kill a bigger dragon for me?"
"That's my duty," the knight replied,
Hoping to get on her better side.
This dragon was big, it breathed real fire.

But this knight was bold and did not tire.

He pierced the belly with his sword.

The dragon died without another breath or word.

So again he brought back the tail and ears,

Hoping to hear the maiden's cheers.

But none came, for she wanted more,

A bigger dragon killed to its core.

Back on his horse the knight did fly,

Straight to the cave where dragons lie.

This was a battle for which songs were written,

About how the dragon was finally smitten.

The dragon, ready to kill, did not see his knife,

And with great skill he took its life.

But the maiden sang not and made one more request.

The knight was done; he wanted no more test,

And off he disappeared, toward the west.

She turned away, and thought she knew best.

He wasn't her white knight, just like the rest.

Many women (and many men, for that matter) have what we call the "White Knight Syndrome" (WKS). Every person they meet is not quite right. Sometimes they know right away that someone is wrong for them. Other times, they go out with a man or even live with him a while before they realize that he is wrong for them. To those with WKS, it seems that "all the good ones are taken."

In truth, however, all those "taken" white knights weren't always white knights. They were frogs, just like all the other guys, until some woman had the wisdom to notice their princely potential and teach them how they wished to be treated.

How do these women teach these frogs to be knights? They train them through being nice, which means that they tell the truth without anger. They also make their men feel like heroes, giving them clear communications until their men succeed at understanding and fulfilling the women's requests. In the saga above, the knight never gets to feel like a hero; he's only a butcher. If the maiden had properly acknowledged him and made him feel that he was winning, he gladly would have continued to slay dragons for her.

We know a woman who has been looking for her knight for the past ten years. One guy was too poor. Another spent too much money and attention on his cars. Another guy was too old. Another was too ugly. Another boyfriend was hooked on porno tapes. One was too politically conservative; another was too into liberal causes. Another had a funny accent. Another had warts on his face (a real frog!). One was too religious. One smoked and drank too much. The list goes on and on.

We don't think that everyone has to be in a couple, but if you say that is something you want, the only way to successfully create a wonderful, nurturing relationship is to find some frog and make him your knight through love and attention. It's a good idea to shop around, of course—you don't have to marry the first frog that comes hopping along, even though some "first love" marriages have lasted and thrived. When, and if, you decide to couple up, you'll have a better sense of what is available. Then you can choose the person who will make the best lifelong companion. By using the training cycle—that is, by using lots of acknowledgment and approval and by not doubting your desire— you will be able to make a white knight out of any frog.

## ⨪ Jealousy ⨪

Although you may have found your prince or princess, that doesn't mean you will live happily ever after. Jealousy can create a lot of problems.

Most people think that jealousy is a negative emotion. Earlier in this book, we explained that emotions are perceived as positive or negative based upon how much responsibility we feel for creating the situation that gave rise to the emotions. With jealousy, obviously, most people feel out of control. This isn't always the case, however. In this section, we will explore the different components of jealousy and explain the best ways that we have found to get a handle on it.

Jealousy is the sum of three parts: envy, exclusion, and tumescence. If you can get rid of exclusion and envy, you will be left with tumescence. This is not so easy, but it can be done. Envy is caused when someone has something that you want, and it drives you crazy. It can be anything from your neighbor having a bigger car than you to your partner flirting with someone else. When you feel envy, you are out of agreement with the way that the world is. To be out of agreement is a sure way to lose; it's a form of being "out of your mind." The easiest way to regain sanity is to get into agreement with the world. Find the world perfect the way that it is and realize that it is okay to want things and that you don't have to let that fact drive you crazy.

What about exclusion? In our society, most relationships are based on serial monogamy. We're supposed to be with one person at a time and have feelings for only that person. Many relationships end, or at least get messy, when one partner doesn't live up to this agreement, the other partner grows jealous, and fighting ensues. People get jealous over both real and imagined sexual acts. They also can get jealous over their partner being romantic with someone else, even if there is no sexual indiscretion. Most people who have affairs or "stray" don't admit it to their partners because they do not wish to be punished for their acts or because they wish to continue their affairs.

When you withhold such an important part of your life from your partner, you like them less. You feel distant from them. The more you withhold, the more distant you become. Your lying and withholding make you lose respect for them, especially if they believe the lies. (Most women know or can intuit when their partner is lying to them, but sometimes they don't want to know for sure, and they keep the relationship going even as it slowly deteriorates.)

To handle the exclusion part of jealousy, include yourself. We know a woman whose husband had an affair with another woman. He did not initially have sex with the woman, but they were very flirtatious and necked in his car. His wife found out through her intuition, which was confirmed by her friends. She was deeply hurt and became very jealous. She decided to confront the other woman, and they met for breakfast at a local restaurant. To her surprise, she found that the other woman wasn't really so bad. In fact, they had a lot in common. They actually became friends, and the wife even set up a date for her husband to have sex with this woman. But it turned out that he didn't have much fun during this "allowed" sex, so the affair ended. The two women stayed friends.

Not all scenarios end so cleanly, of course. Yet it's still in your best interest to include yourself if you feel excluded. It's also wise to own up to the fact that you're jealous. Some people refuse to admit their jealousy, even to themselves. They are either lying or totally numb. Would you want a partner who never felt or showed any jealousy to you, no matter what you did? Some people keep raising the stakes if their partner won't admit their jealousy. To say that you're jealous without being angry or vindictive is a way to show your love. Admitting your jealousy won't make the relationship that is making you jealous go away, but at least you are demonstrating your true feelings and your love.

Woody Allen said, "God gave man a brain and a penis, but only enough blood to operate one at a time." This does not mean that men are guiltless when they stray. Everyone is responsible for his or her life. Men usually stray for lust, as the fun at home is probably absent, while women have affairs when they feel neglected and some man offers them romance. In many cultures, men have wives and mistresses. Our culture frowns upon extramarital sex, so it is up to the couple to keep the communication lines open and keep the fun going in the relationship. If people are afraid to share their deepest thoughts and desires with their partners for fear of punishment, they are probably doomed to either a dull relationship or one that is challenged by adultery.

What you are left with, once you have removed envy and exclusion, is tumescence, the sexual energy that can be used for great orgasms. This heightened energy is too strong for many people to handle pleasurably, and that is why a lot of people fight to bring the energy down to a more comfortable level before they have sex. If you can channel this energy into pleasure at its highest point, you will be amazed. Jealousy has been now turned into a positive emotion.

Many people live their lives as victims. They do not take responsibility for creating their lives as they would like to live them. By waiting for the white knight to show up and make their lives wonderful, they are relinquishing their responsibility to outside forces. They are setting themselves up to lose. People also become victims when confronted with jealousy. Unless they take responsibility for their jealousy, they will suffer. By being responsible for your life and all of its emotions, you can create a life that you appreciate and value.

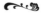

# CHAPTER 12

# Safe Sex

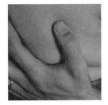

*B*ecause any sexual activity, including EMO techniques, can expose you to sexually transmitted diseases (STDs), we've included this chapter, which will discuss how to keep yourself and your partner safe. We will discuss human immunodeficiency virus (HIV) and acquired immune deficiency syndrome (AIDS, which results from HIV) and explain the best ways to avoid getting HIV while still having lots of pleasure. We will also describe other STDs and explain how genital injury can be prevented by paying attention during sexual activity.

## ✐ HIV and AIDS ❧

When Vera and I started exploring and researching sex in the late 1960s and early 1970s, there was no such thing as HIV or AIDS. There were other STDs, such as gonorrhea and syphilis, but no one was particularly concerned with safety during sex, because those diseases were curable. Lots of folks (especially in California) had lots of sex with lots of different partners. But with the advent of HIV and AIDS in the 1980s, all that changed.

Now, there is no completely safe form of sex, except for masturbation, phone sex, and cybersex. Health clinics and sex-study courses in schools recommend that men use condoms whenever they have intercourse with anyone who isn't their monogamous partner. In addition, dental dams (special devices that can be used while performing fellatio or cunnilingus) are recommended. We've known some students who used Saran Wrap as a dental dam. Condoms and dams are safer than not using anything, but they are still a form of Russian roulette. They can break or leak, and this does happen a small percentage of the time. If you wish to have sex that involves any swapping of mucus or other bodily fluids, such as semen or vaginal secretions, we urge you to take all necessary precautions to prevent transmission of HIV and other STDs.

Besides vaginal intercourse, anal sex is extremely risky, because this form of penetration can easily cause abrasion and bleeding. Supposedly, unprotected anal sex was responsible for the high rate of gay men contracting HIV in the 1980s. Even kissing may involve some risk (although there are few, if any, cases of HIV transmission via kissing): for example, if both partners have bleeding gums. Be careful—it's your life.

The onslaught of AIDS dampened the sexual exuberance of the 1960s and 1970s, which was already slowing due to the ordinary cycles that sexuality goes through in society, from repression to openness and back again. (For example, the eighteenth century was relatively open sexually, but the Victorian era was more repressed—people even put skirts on table legs to prevent men from thinking about sex!). Because of this natural cycle, society probably will become more open about sex once again in the coming years. It's our hope that "doing" will be the first choice of responsible people. "Doing," especially the practice of artful clitoral stimulation, is one of the safer forms of sexual activity (in addition to being among the more orgasmically gratifying). Nobody gets pregnant from it, and there's hardly any chance of contracting an STD.

## ⟿ Other Sexually ⟿
## Transmitted Diseases

Most STDs are transmitted through intercourse. These include bacterial infections such as gonorrhea, syphilis, chlamydia (which is the most common STD), and gardnerella. Genital warts and herpes, as well as HIV, are viral infections. Trichimonas, a protozoan infection, can be spread through intercourse and even through sharing a towel. Candidiasis, or yeast infection, can also be contracted through intercourse. Many of these diseases produce a similar set of symptoms in women, such as extra discharge, a foul odor, and even vaginal bleeding. Men can get enlarged testicles or feel a burning sensation during urination. However, often these STDs do not manifest any symptoms, especially in men, for an extended period and thus can go unnoticed until they cause damage. If you are single and have had previous sexual partners, we recommend that you ask a doctor to check you and any future partner for all STDs before you commence any sexual activity that involves an exchange of bodily fluids. Meanwhile, you can have a lot of fun with latex and, especially, with doing.

## ⟿ Latex ⟿

The chances of spreading HIV or other STDs through doing are very remote. To prevent even that tiny chance from becoming a reality, however, we recommend that people who have not been tested for HIV—especially those who have had other recent sexual partners—use latex gloves when doing each other. This is because the "doer" might have a cut finger, and they will be touching the bodily fluids of the "doee." There are other ways of transmitting HIV and other STDs besides mucus exchange, such as blood transfusions and sharing needles. And, sadly, people do lie about their sex lives, so unless you really know someone, you should assume that either they could lie or could have been lied to by one of their past partners. So unless you're completely certain of your partner, latex is your best choice for protection. It is always better to err on the side of safety.

We recommend using thin surgical gloves. You can buy them at almost any drugstore. We have used many different brands, and you can experiment to see which brand fits and feels best to you. When you put on the gloves, make sure the fingertips are smoothed and that any bubbles of air caught beneath the gloves are removed before you touch your partner.

With the gloves, you'll want to use a lubricant. In the past, we recommended using a water-soluble lubricant containing 5 percent nonoxynol-9, which is supposed to be antiviral, with latex gloves. However, further studies have shown that nonoxynol-9 actually causes skin abrasions, so we no longer recommend it. There are many water-soluble lubricants on the market today that are fine with latex. Any petroleum-based lubricant should be avoided when using latex, as it tends to break the latex down. That goes for condoms as well as latex gloves.

We have found that after you get used to using latex gloves that fit you well, you do not notice the difference between your naked hand and a gloved hand. The person getting done might even prefer the latex, as they won't have to feel calluses or sharp fingernails. (If one is serious about becoming a doing artist, the nails must be kept very short and smooth, whether one uses gloves or not.) When you use latex gloves with a new partner, it demonstrates your integrity to them and gives them one more reason to surrender. You really are showing respect for them and for yourself. At the height of the AIDS scare, we even used two sets of gloves with nonoxynol-9 between the gloves. Then when we removed one set of gloves, the hand felt like it was naked.

## ✍ Genital Injury ✍

Our genitals are made of very strong and durable tissue. When proper lubrication is used, they can be rubbed and stroked for many hours without any injury. When injury does occur, it is because of inattention (and perhaps covert anger). Paying attention can help to prevent injuries such as chafed penises and banged cervixes.

We have noticed that when women get infections, either genital or urinary-tract infections, after intercourse, it usually occurs because they had sex when they didn't feel like it and thus weren't sufficiently lubricated. Abrasion can also happen if either the bodily lubrication or externally applied lubrication wears off. Some people are macho and refuse to add lubrication because they feel that it should be naturally supplied, and any application of lubricant makes them feel like failures. This is silly thinking and only gets them into trouble. When doing for long periods of time, it is of the utmost importance to keep genital tissue well lubricated.

When women pass menopause, their ability to self-lubricate usually decreases. When post-menopausal women have intercourse, it's an especially good idea for their partners to add some lubricant to their erect cocks before insertion.

There are many lubricants on the market, and you can check them out until you find one that feels good and is compatible with your body. Applying a water-soluble lubricant to genitals is a lot of fun. It feels great going on. However, lubricant can get sticky after continued stroking. You can add some water to the already applied lubricant to make it feel fresh and slick again. When we use a water-soluble lubricant like KY Jelly, we keep a glass of water nearby to dip our fingers into when the lubricant gets sticky. This not only feels a lot better than adding more lubricant, but also saves some money, because you don't have to buy lots of lubricant. When you're doing a man's cock with water-soluble lubricant, you can use a spray bottle filled with water to reduce stickiness and refresh the lubricant.

As we have described, there are many sexually transmitted diseases that you could come into contact with during sexual activity. But by being responsible and choosing to take proper precautions, you can limit your and your partner's risk of infection. This demonstrates integrity to your partner, which allows them to trust you more, surrender to your touch, and experience more intense EMOs.

# Conclusion

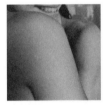

**W**e have come down far enough. We now invite you to take the information that you have received from this book and use it to make your life more pleasurable. Before we leave you, however, we'd like to close with some thoughts about how to go for what you really want—a lifetime of intense pleasure and joy.

## ✒ You Can't Avoid Bad ✑

There is no way to avoid bad things. In fact, as soon as you form a conception that something is bad, that thing has some existence in your life. It's like trying not to think of pink elephants. Your universe is composed of the things that you place your attention on.

Putting your attention on avoiding the bad is a sure way to lose. When football teams are winning a game with aggressive play and then change their focus to what they call a "prevent" defense, you know that they are in trouble. The other team will soon be right back in the game. They are trying to avoid the bad, and just the use of the word *try* indicates probable failure. If all your attention is focused on losing, the best you can hope for is a zero-zero score at the end of the game. To use another analogy, when the captain in *Star Trek* commands that all energy be directed into the shields, there's no way that the crew can defeat their enemies. All they can hope for is a standoff.

In our sensual lives, when we try to avoid the bad, what we actually avoid is experience. Experience includes the bad, but it also includes the good. Rather than face rejection, many people don't take any risks and don't ask for what they like. For example, they might not make a sensual offer. They wind up alone or they don't get to do something that they would have enjoyed, but at least they weren't rejected. The choice is really between feeling and numbness, not between good and bad.

## ✒ Buy a Ticket ✑

If you want to win, the best way to accomplish it is to go for the good. Go ahead and make that offer. Then do what it takes to reach your goals pleasurably. If you want to win the lottery, you have to buy a ticket. If you want to have a wonderful life, one with many experiences, you have to risk playing the game of life.

In any game, there's the possibility of losing. However, as many enlightened beings have stated, it's the path that counts (or "It's how you play the game that matters"). You can learn something from each loss or failure and use that lesson to win the next time you play. If you stay at home and never make offers, you may not be rejected, but you will also never get to win. Use your new seduction abilities to help yourself pleasurably overcome resistance or obstacles. You can choose to see the obstacles in your life as resistance that you can enjoy overcoming. Games are problems that we enjoy, and problems are games that we deny wanting to play. Problems exist because people refuse to see the solution, even if it is obvious to someone else. People become attached to their problems. In our work, we have found that when a student clings to a problem, it's best not to try to remove it but to give the student a new, more enjoyable problem to concentrate upon.

## Spontaneous Deliberate Pleasure

Our society pressures us to believe that sensual pleasure should be spontaneous, that we shouldn't have to plan it. We think that if you have not planned to create pleasure and fun in your life, there's a good chance that they may never happen. The more you plan for them, the more they'll happen.

If you have young children, as a number of our friends do, and you're waiting for the spontaneous fun genie to appear, you'll wait a long time. You have to plan specific times and places where you can deliberately have pleasurable sensual experiences. This goes for people without small children, too. The more you plan and train for fun by teaching your own body and teaching your partner how you like to be touched and pleasured, the more spontaneous pleasure you will experience.

## Go For It!

We hope that you'll use the information in this book to turn yourself on. We hope that you'll also use it to find someone (a new friend or someone whom you already know) to have fun with, teaching them how to pleasure you and learning how to pleasure them. Do your sensuality exercises frequently, if possible.

Your life can be enhanced, refreshed, and expanded if you learn more about your own body. If you learn about your partner's sensual feelings and thoughts and openly express your own, you will open yourself up to the possibilities of a wonderful relationship, one with more intimacy than you have ever had or even thought possible. We think that once you are on the path to realizing your full sensual potential and are becoming more orgasmic, the rest of your life will become better as well. You will be nicer. You will be more generous. You will be more joyous in your day-to-day life. You might live longer, not to mention more healthily. You might even become more aware of your spirituality. The choice is yours, and we encourage you to *go for it!*

# *Appendix A*

## COMMONLY ASKED
## QUESTIONS AND ANSWERS

We have found that some questions are asked over and over again in our courses about orgasm, so we have included this appendix of questions and answers for your use while you study EMO.

Q How can I touch my girlfriend directly on her clitoris if she finds it too sensitive to be touched?

A Many women have never touched their own clitorises, let alone had someone else touch them. We have met many women who thought at first that their clitorises were too sensitive to be touched, but all eventually learned to love having their clitorises directly stroked. Your partner could have had a negative experience in the past: Perhaps a guy who did not know what he was doing touched her clitoris with too much pressure and hurt her.

Touching someone directly on her clitoris who has never had it done before can be very scary to her. When you touch her, you have to do so with confidence and direct communication.

A hood covers the clitoris. This hood is sometimes thin, sometimes thick, and we've even met a couple of women whose clitoral hoods were so attached to their clitorises that they could not be pulled back and up. This is a very rare condition, however, and even those women were able to experience intense orgasm by rubbing directly on their hoods.

When touching a woman for the first time, tell her what you will do before you do it. First, put a glob of lubricant on her clitoris. Then pull the hood back with either your free hand or the thumb of your "doing" hand. We suggest that at first you touch her with only the lubricant; let your finger touch the lubricant but not her skin. This can be a lot of fun, and if it's done playfully and intentionally, she will probably feel safe enough that you can eventually touch her skin with increasing pressure.

Start with a very light touch, so that your partner can ask for more pressure. If you start with too firm a touch, she will back away from you and put more energy toward defending herself. The goal now, as always, is to have the touch feel good at each moment. You are in no rush to get to any specific place or act.

*Q* What can I do to have my husband pay more attention to me?

*A* To attract someone, you have to be attractive. To be adored by someone, you have to be adorable. Men are success junkies. They love to win. They love producing for women. The best way to get a man and keep him is to have him win with you. The easiest way to have him win is to be happy and have him be responsible for your happiness. Once he feels like a winner around you, his addiction to success will keep him very attentive toward you.

This is more difficult than it sounds for many women, because they may feel anger toward men in general. Basically, you have to decide what is more important to you, happiness or anger. When a man feels that there is no way to win with you, or if he feels like a loser, he becomes apathetic. This apathy is demonstrated by lack of attention and by not listening to you.

To gain his attention, you will have to become a lot nicer, which means a lot happier, which means giving up your anger. Men can be quite dumb, so don't expect him to hear what you want the first time. You may have to repeat the communication a number of times before he gets it. This is best done by repeating the communication in the same way each time until he's gotten it. If you change the way you phrase it, you will probably only confuse him. Once he does get it, let him know that he's winning, and you will have the beginnings of a trained man.

**Q** How can I keep my lover from going over the edge and then not wanting to be touched anymore?

**A** This question is from a man but could very well be from a woman. The dictionary defines *orgasm* as the climax of sexual tension. This is a very limiting definition: It describes the usual male ejaculatory orgasm that goes tense, tense, tense, and then squirt, squirt, squirt. You will have to reeducate or recondition yourself as well as your lover to relax rather than tense. Every time she tenses, gently tell her to relax. You can tell her to push out, which helps people relax; when they tense up, they are usually pulling in. Then continue rubbing until you think the next stroke or two will put her over the edge, and then peak her. After she comes down slightly, you can continue your stroking. The pleasurable feeling that she is having is really orgasm, and as long as you keep peaking her and she doesn't tense up, she will continue to be able to be touched. Each of her peaks will eventually become more intense than her old way of coming. Reread the section on peaking in Chapter 7.

**Q** What can I do to have my husband talk to me more?

**A** This is very similar to the question on page 174 in which a woman asked how to get a man to put more attention on her. Verbally, men are usually duller than women. You might want to spend some time with your girlfriends when you want livelier conversations, but if the attention you want from him is oral, give him lots of rewards for any talking that he *does* do. Don't beat him up for being the strong, silent type, because that's the way he was conditioned. Just recondition him with lots of wins and positive reinforcement. A man who feels like a winner around you will do anything you ask, even talk more.

*Q* What do women want?

*A* Different women want different things, but a woman basically wants to be the priority in your life. She wants your attention first and foremost. She wants to be loved and cared for. After attention (which includes sex), she wants her necessities taken care of, and then she wants pleasurable things, which (depending on the woman) could include shared activities like sports or luxury gifts like jewelry. Some women who are not getting enough of their partners' attention will settle for jewelry and other baubles, but they won't be as happy as their sisters who get lots of attention. Women will notice the areas in which you hold out on them, and they'll want you to give that particular thing to them. A smart woman is someone who wants a lot and who makes you feel like you want to give her that and more.

Women also order short, which means that they want to be overwhelmed. They may say they want a nineteen-inch television, but perhaps they really want a large, thirty-six-inch screen. She may also order short by category, saying that she wants to go out to eat, but perhaps she really would like you to have sex with her, then make or get her favorite food and feed it to her in bed. You can tell if that is something she wants by how her face lights up when you bring up the idea. We call this technique "presenting her with a menu." Watch her face as you mention different types of restaurants. How about Japanese, Chinese, or Italian food? How about getting done before dinner?

This does not mean that women do not like to get, or cannot get, things for themselves. It does mean that when women's wants and desires are fulfilled and appreciated, their relationships with men are happy and highly functional. It means that both parties win. A woman may want something that a man does not think he can get or produce for her, but if he feels true desire, the energy to fulfill the want will come with the order. He may be surprised and pleased with himself if he does something that he never thought he could do.

*Q* How can I enjoy his cock more?

*A* The first thing you have to do is to enjoy your pussy. You can do this with your exercises and by getting done. Only play with his cock when you want to, not when you think you should or because you feel guilty.

His cock can be a really fun toy to play with. When touched with enjoyment, it responds with enthusiasm and salutes your femininity. Touch it to have your hand, mouth, or pussy feel pleasure. You can also create training sessions in which you explore a cock visually. First, re-read Chapter 8's information on training from cause, focusing on the techniques for putting your partner at ease and making him feel safe. Then take the cock in your hands and look at it from all sides. Then smell and taste it from all sides.

Next, experiment with different pressures and strokes that may feel good to your partner. Remember to ask before you squeeze harder, and proceed in small increments. When the cock is engorged, it will be able to take more pressure. You may have more fun playing with his cock if you are coming or have come already. Check out the "Coming Together" section in Chapter 9.

When you do him, manually or orally, remember that the only goal is to have each moment, each stroke, feel great. Don't feel under pressure to make him squirt. He will anyway, if the pleasure is there. Only fuck when you really want to. If you become good at having EMOs, you will be able to have an orgasm practically at will. When doing his cock, you can feel your pussy and experience your own orgasm as you take him for a ride.

*Q* Should we talk business when we are making out?

*A* We would not recommend that. A better idea is to talk about it afterward (but not too soon afterward). At that point, both of you, hopefully, will be detumesced and thinking a lot more clearly than before you made out.

After experiencing intense orgasm, things look more beautiful, food tastes better, and the world is a better place.

*Q* Why do you say that men don't get their own cocks hard?

*A* We belong to the family of animals known as mammals (named after the mammary glands). The way sex happens in mammals is that the female goes into heat and then the male tries to copulate with her, using, of course, his hard cock. The penis is really a sack that fills with blood when the male is stimulated. Just as salivation is a physical response caused by food, hard cocks are a response caused by a female in heat.

Of course, humans as well as animals can be conditioned to produce a physical response when encountering signals other than the primary one—for example, Pavlov's dogs salivated in response to a bell. Humans can fantasize about a female in heat or even some event to which they have a conditioned response. Every time there's a hard cock, there isn't necessarily a female in heat; however, there often is. We have heard many men complain that they cannot always get their cocks hard when they want to and that they get hard when they don't want to. Female humans have the power to turn on men at will. Men can sometimes get their own cocks hard when they masturbate or have homosexual sex, or sometimes even when they are with a woman.

When we say that men don't get their cocks hard, what we are really saying is that the primary source of the erection is the woman. The lesson for men is to understand that they don't have to worry about getting hard and that the woman can get it hard, if she has true use for it, at any time. He should not blame himself or his partner, and he can do something else that is fun and does not require a hard cock. There are, of course, some men with severe vascular disease that impairs their ability to get hard, and they should seek professional help.

*Q* Is it okay for my boyfriend to do me if he isn't turned on?

*A* Yes. He has to want to touch you and give you pleasure, but a hard cock is not necessary to do you. In order for you to have the best orgasm possible, you must both place your attention on you. This does not mean that he *shouldn't* be turned on, only that it is not necessary. When I do Vera in our one-hour DEMO, my cock may not be hard for part of or even the whole hour. This does not mean that I am not having a fantastic time pleasuring her. It only means that our thoughts are not on my having a hard cock at those times. We have taught some physiologically impotent men to do their lovers, and it really made them feel like potent men again, able to give their lovers more pleasure than they ever could before, even when they were young and healthy. If you worry about whether he is turned on, your attention is not on your coming, and your orgasm will be lessened. If you relax and enjoy yourself to the fullest, don't be surprised if his cock does get hard.

*Q* Why do I take so long to start coming?

*A* Your attention is on some future event, some potential orgasm that you want to reach but have not reached yet. That is why, in our masturbation exercise in Chapter 5, we insisted that you not do it for the future orgasm, but for the pleasure that you feel with each stroke. Most people have been conditioned to believe that orgasm looks like the typical male ejaculation. That is a very limiting viewpoint, a sexual prejudice that you can recondition. Orgasm is the natural state, and you must have non-confronted it in order to not feel it. To experience orgasm, all you need to do is just feel the pleasure at the moment and realize that you are coming on the first stroke. As a matter of fact, you don't even have to be stroked to have an orgasm. People have wet dreams all the time. All you need to do is have your genitals feel better than any other part of your body. It is really about rearranging your attitudes and knowing that many people were once in the same place that you are and are now having EMOs.

*Q* Why do I come so fast when I fuck my girlfriend, and what can I do about it?

*A* There are a number of reasons that men have premature ejaculations: They may be young or inexperienced, worried about their performance, or too horny, or perhaps their girlfriends want only a little bit of them. But there is something that you can do about it.

If you become adept at doing her before you have intercourse, much of the pressure to perform during intercourse is removed. When you do have intercourse, you can't prematurely ejaculate, as she has already had an orgasm for an extended time. Whenever you come will be just fine, and because the pressure has been removed, it is likely that your ejaculation won't be as hasty as before. We don't recommend doing what Woody Allen describes himself doing, thinking about Willy Mays sliding into home plate to prevent ejaculation or thinking about depressing topics to keep yourself from coming. You might, if you're too horny, masturbate before having intercourse in order to last longer. But we also strongly recommend rubbing on your girlfriend's clitoris before intercourse, as it is just as important for the woman to be engorged as it is for the man. She will enjoy the intercourse much more, and she might not want to get it over with so quickly.

*Q* What can I do to get a man and have him treat me the way I want?

*A* This is really the same question that was asked earlier: How can I get my husband to pay more attention to me? Basically, you have to be nicer than anyone else is to him. You have to be attractive and turn him on. Men are not used to winning with women, so when a woman finally finds a man "right," he wants to spend more time with her.

You don't want to chase or crowbar him into wanting you. You want to be so irresistible that he cannot resist you and chases you. Sex appeal has very little to do with a person's actual looks, but it does have a lot to do with the way you feel about yourself, how turned on you are to yourself. The mirror exercise in Chapter 5 is an excellent way to turn yourself on.

Once you turn him on and let him know that he's winning with you, it also helps to give him tasks at which he can succeed. Men are great at goal achievement but poor at goal selection. You can help him with this, getting him to do things that he didn't think he could achieve. With your turn-on and support, he is able to accomplish these goals. This is a way for men to reach glory and become heroes. Sometimes, women doubt their own attractiveness and are afraid to ask men for things because they feel that the men won't want to do things for them. But it is remarkable how much men can produce with just a little encouragement. If they win, they will be yours forever.

We knew a couple in which the man was quite attractive yet doubted his ability to produce. He was a go-fer for an investment firm, getting coffee and doughnuts and other supplies for the brokers and investment counselors. His wife was not especially beautiful, but she liked herself and had a lot of faith in her husband. She encouraged him to take the test to become a broker, and after he passed the exam, he started work on the bottom rung of his company. Within five years he was vice-president of the company and making close to seven figures. They have two children, a big house, and a live-in nanny, and they're devoted to each other and their children. Indeed, they're a very happy couple, and the wife's encouragement was a key element in their success.

*Q* Does the size of a man's cock matter?

*A* It may matter to his self-image, but it has no effect on how much sensation his lover feels during intercourse. When a woman's genitals are engorged and pushed out, even a small appendage feels quite large inside her. During our DEMO, after I have rubbed on Vera for some time, I insert just the tip of my thumb into her introitus. She experiences the sensation almost to her navel. This proves that size does not matter to a woman who is turned on and engorged.

Also, remember that penises range from those that have a large coefficient of expansion (in other words, they're small when flaccid but grow significantly in erection) to those that get only slightly larger upon engorgement. A man's penis may be very small when flaccid but grow into a huge organ when engorged. The size and shape of a penis also change according to who is enjoying it and how much cock she wants to have for that particular sexual act.

Many men are extremely sensitive in this area (pardon the pun). If they believe their penises are too small, they are embarrassed and shy around women or may suffer even worse neuroses. Again, the hand is a much more efficient way to give a woman an extended orgasm than the penis. In fact, a small hand can actually be an advantage in reaching her spot and playing with her clitoris.

On the other hand, if the cock is larger than normal, most vaginas are usually able to handle it. It is a good idea to lubricate the penis before insertion, even if the woman is usually lubricated, as a small dry area could cause abrasion. Some people think that it is "wrong" to use lubricant before intercourse; we don't. As a woman gets older, she tends to lubricate less than she did when she was younger, so it is especially important for post-menopausal women. It is always important that the woman as well as the man be engorged before intercourse.

*Q* What do you think about Viagra?

*A* We think that when it is used properly, it can enhance the sexual experience. However, the emphasis of our work is on producing better orgasms for women. We feel that the best lover is the one who can produce the most pleasure. To become an artist in doing makes a man an extremely valuable commodity. A flaccid penis can be stroked and feel wonderful sensations, so a hard penis is unnecessary to either give or receive pleasure.

Many men are psychologically impotent. If they learn how to pleasure a woman with their hands, however, they'll feel better about themselves, and the women they are with might even be able to engorge their cocks without Viagra. However, for men who are physiologically impotent due to circulation problems, and who have learned to pleasure women by hand, we think Viagra could be useful.

*Q* What is the best way to have sex with more than two people?

*A* *Menages à trois* can be a lot of fun, but they're very tricky to pull off. They should be settings in which everyone wins, which can be hard to arrange. We think that the best threesomes happen among two women and one man (although if all three partners are willing participants, it doesn't really matter what sex they are). Two men and one woman is a feasible arrangement, too, but the second man doesn't add much to the equation; two women, on the other hand, can turn each other on as well as turning on the man. In addition, many women are more open to having sex with other women than men are about having sex with other men. Regardless of the partners' sexes, however, all the participants should like one another, and the communication has to be top-notch.

*Q* Is oral sex as effective as doing for giving a woman an orgasm?

*A* We think that oral sex is a wonderful way of giving and receiving pleasure. Like all sex acts, however, the person performing cunnilingus has to
be licking and sucking for their own pleasure. Oral sex is very erotic and,
if done effectively, can be lots of fun.

Remember, however, that eroticism comes from breaking minor social taboos.
It is like adding a spice to a meal. It can enhance the taste and pleasure of the
meal, but on its own it is not very nutritious. Oral sex and other erotic acts
have to be the spice, not the main meal. That means that the communication
from the person being sucked and licked has to be very specific, as it is very
difficult to talk with your mouth full of pussy. It can also be a difficult skill to
hone: it's hard to get visual confirmation of what your tongue and mouth are
actually doing. To illustrate this issue, we usually ask people in our classes
whether they would prefer a brain surgeon to use his hands or tongue when
operating on them.

Oral sex can be lots of fun, especially when the partners have great communication and experience each stroke; however, when it comes to effective-
ness or efficiency in producing an orgasm, the first choice is manual stimulation. Once a person learns their way around a pussy and becomes an actual
doing artist, their ability to perform cunnilingus also improves.

*Q* I had this really wonderful and intense orgasm with my boyfriend about
one year ago. How can I duplicate that experience?

*A* You can't duplicate that experience. Each orgasm is different, and
the experience depends on many factors. When your attention is focused
on comparing your present orgasm to one that happened in the past,
your attention, obviously, is not on what you're feeling now. To have an

optimal orgasm, you must keep your total attention on what you presently feel.

An excellent way to stay present with your orgasm is to verbally acknowledge any pleasurable sensations that you feel. You don't have to think of fancy things to say; simple words such as "yes" or "that feels good" are okay. The more specific the acknowledgment, the better. Specific acknowledgments, such as "That light stroke on my clitoris feels electric," are great and will get you higher as well as keep you focused.

*Q* How do I get my new boyfriend to rub me more lightly?

*A* By being nice and telling him the truth about what you want, without anger. Before he starts touching you, you can touch him on his arm or on the back of his hand, demonstrating how much pressure you would like him to use. You can let him know that you like different pressures and will let him know when you would like more or less pressure. On your own body, you can show him where you like to be touched and what kind of stroke you prefer.

Teach him to use the taking touch. Have him touch you as he would touch silk or velvet, things that he touches in order to make his hand feel wonderful. Our hands are an essential part of being human, and they've enabled us to reach the top of the mammalian world. Our hands can do so many different things, from building tools and machines to pulling out a splinter. They can be used and treated as sexual body parts when touching for pleasure. Be sure to have him take good care of his hands. Ensure his hands are manicured regularly (by a professional, by himself, or by you). Nails must be short, with smooth corners, if you desire him to be an artist in sensual pleasure. Have him moisturize his hands frequently to keep them soft. If he has bad calluses or really rough hands, you can suggest that he consider using a latex glove for smoothness. It's mostly the tip of his finger that he uses, so the roughness of the rest of his hand is not usually a problem.

In his previous relationships with women, your boyfriend may have been trained or conditioned to use a strong touch. Or perhaps he has never used his hands on a pussy before and he just doesn't know any better. In either case, you can teach him to touch you with the perfect touch if you communicate with him. The person who communicates something is responsible for making sure that the recipient hears and understands what is communicated. This might mean that you have to repeat the instruction more than once to get through to him. If you worry about hurting his feelings by doing this, you might lie there without talking and quickly start to resent his incompetent touch. This might make you less nice. It might be helpful to re-read the section on training from effect in Chapter 8.

## Appendix B

### A DAY OF PLEASURE AND ATTENTION

The following is a description of one way to thoroughly pleasure someone you know intimately, and with whom you have been doing sensual training. It is something that you may want to do in its totality on special occasions, such as Valentine's Day or your lover's birthday. It is not something that most people will do regularly. However, small sections of what follows can be used more frequently.

Remember that this is just one example, and you can tailor the experience however you would like. Some people think that you shouldn't deliberately plan pleasure, that it should happen naturally. We think that it is great to deliberately plan sensual experiences and that if you do, you will experience more unplanned fun as well.

The example that we show here is of a man putting his attention on a woman. But women can also use these ideas on men. When a woman does this for a man, the major difference is that she takes care of her own tumescence before she takes care of his. Also, depending on the man, she may want to limit the time she spends teasing his body.

## The Tumescence Starts

After sleeping peacefully in bed together, they awaken. He looks into her eyes and tells her how beautiful she is. He tells her that she needs no makeup or grooming, that she is a natural beauty. She smiles. He takes her hand and gently kisses it. (When you touch or kiss someone, remember to use a touch and a kiss that feels good to you. You are not trying to make an impression on them.)

Softly squeezing her hand, he gazes at her and tells her that when he comes home from work in the afternoon, he will pleasure every part of her body and give her the best orgasm she has ever had. She doesn't answer right away. As he continues to look at her with admiration and love, she answers that that would be wonderful.

As soon as she agrees to the future experience, the tumescence starts to build. He asks if he may kiss her, and she agrees to that. He places his lips softly against her lips, holding the back of her head with his hands, making her feel loved and surrounded. He moves his lips slowly, letting his tongue touch the inside of her lips without penetrating her mouth. The kiss lasts about thirty seconds, and they both feel it all over their bodies. He releases his hands and lips and lets her know that he feels aroused but now will get out of bed and remember that kiss forever. The tumescence builds some more.

After showering and dressing, they eat breakfast together. He has squeezed some fresh orange juice, and with it he toasts her beauty and how wonderful his life is because of her. They kiss again. She wants to take him back to bed, yet with much difficulty he resists his lust so he can give her even more pleasure later. He lets her know how he feels. (She is also testing him at this point by seeing if she can take back control and if he is indeed serious about this great orgasm later.) They have a passionate hug at the front door, with their entire bodies pressing against each other, and he gives her one more sweet kiss.

## Teasing

He leaves for the day. Later in the morning, she finds a poem that he has left for her:

> I will touch you oh so sweet
> From your head to your feet
> Your soul will itself meet
> As I play your special heat
> I know where you hide

And where you wish to go
I will take you for a ride
And stop before you know
I will have you come toward me
Make you beg while you defend
I shall have you angels see
I will tease you to the end.

He calls her around lunchtime, says one word—"tonight"—and then hangs up. The tumescence builds some more.

In the early afternoon, the doorbell rings. When she opens the door, a bouquet of roses and irises (her favorite flowers) are handed to her, with a sweet note saying how much he loves her. She is overwhelmed. The tumescence is still building.

## Preparations

He takes off work early so that he can get everything ready for the special date. He picks up some of her favorite vanilla-scented candles. He picks up CDs by her current favorite musicians. He buys dark-chocolate truffles, raspberries, and the sushi that she loves. He also gets some Pellegrino water and a book of erotic stories. (You need to remember what the person whom you are pleasuring is pleasured by. Not everyone likes sushi, of course—this is only an example. And because you will be at this event, too, make sure that there are things that you like to eat, music that both of you enjoy, and fragrances that you also enjoy smelling.)

## Getting Ready for Anything

He gets home. He remembers that the symptoms of a woman in heat can include irritability. He is hoping for the best, but he's prepared for anything. It is likely that when he walks in the door, a wild woman will meet him. There could be broken appliances, leaky plumbing, and crying children (if they have children).

She greets him at the door with a wild look. He tells her how beautiful she is when she's looking wild and gives her a big hug, this time to bring her down a level. She starts telling him about all the problems she has. With total attention, he listens to everything she has to say. He promises to take care of everything. He is her hero and he is there for her only. He postpones as many of the problems as he can, as they will magically disappear once she comes down. If there is anything that has to be done immediately, he does it (if a pipe is broken, for example, he shuts off the water in that area).

## Back in the Bedroom

He quickly sets up the bedroom with all the fun things that he has gotten for her. She has put the flowers in a vase, and he brings those into the bedroom, too. He lights the candles and gets into comfortable clothes. He puts a "do not disturb" sign on their door. He turns off the telephone ringer and turns down the answering machine. He gets her into the bedroom and closes the door. He looks at her and lets her know how beautiful he finds her.

## Loving Touches

He tells her that he is going to remove all of her outer clothes. He sits her at the edge of the bed and removes her shoes and socks. He kisses her feet. He unbuttons her blouse and slowly removes it, one sleeve at a time. He kisses her hands and arms, letting her know how silky her skin is and how wonderful she smells. He helps her off with her pants and continues to acknowledge her beauty and sexiness. He kisses her calves and thighs and helps her lie down on the bed. He tells her that she has great legs and that her thighs are so beautiful and smooth. He loves her muscle tone, and her thighs really turn him on (most women find their thighs wrong and too big and love hearing how sexy and pretty they are).

She is wearing only a bra and panties now. He tells her that he is going to touch her all over her body, starting from her extremities, her toes, hands, and head, and that his final destination is her pussy. (Even though they know each other, it is still a good idea for him to tell her what he will do before he does it. Surprises are detumescing and will bring her down.) He offers her a bite to eat. He has put a flexible straw in her drink, so she can drink without getting up.

He lightly touches her right foot with a pleasurable stroke that is fairly quick, using his whole hand. He creates focal points on her foot and teases those areas (he doesn't want to massage her with firm pressure, as that will ground her and bring her down, and his intention is to bring her up as high as she can go.) He then does the same for her left foot. He is constantly telling her how beautiful and sexy she is, how much fun she is to touch, and how wonderful her skin feels.

He then goes to her hands and creates focal points there as well, teasing her with the backs of his nails as well as his palm, using quick circular strokes that take her higher. He does the other hand. He then goes to her head and lightly touches her face. With one finger, he gently touches her lips, tumescing them; as they get fuller and redder, he reports what he sees to her. He stays at her lips for a good while, as they are so much fun to touch. He tickles her ears and neck until she can hardly take it anymore.

He then connects all the areas that he has touched so far, and as he goes back to her feet, he brushes her pubic hair through her panties. He turns her over onto her tummy, puts his hand gently on her back, and creates more focal points. He undoes her bra strap and lightly scratches her with the back of his nails. After stroking her back and letting her know how gorgeous her back is, he turns her over again. They each have a bite of chocolate. He kisses her sweet lips.

He removes her bra completely and strokes her chest, using her nipples as focal points. He tells her that her nipples are engorging and getting firm, that her breasts are beautiful and sexy. He then goes back to her ankles and calves and tells her how he loves her calves, how sexy and shapely they are. He touches them lovingly, with light strokes up and down and around, first the right and then the left.

He then connects all the areas that he has touched so far with a quick, loving stroke. He plays with soft touches on her belly, using circular strokes with her navel as the focal point. He tells her he is saving her thighs for next-to-last.

They have some more chocolate before he touches her thighs. First, he slowly removes her panties. He tells her that just thinking of her thighs gets him hard. He starts with her right thigh, stroking up and down with long strokes, reaching almost to her pubic hair and then back toward her knee. He also uses circular strokes, using the upper middle of her inner thigh as the focal point, rubbing first in smaller and smaller circles, then in larger and larger circles, and back to smaller ones. He sniffs her pussy and tells her how ecstatic her scent makes him feel. He then does the same to her left thigh. He deliberately touches her pubic hair lightly with the back of his hand, just one touch, and lets her know that he will get there soon, but not quite yet.

## Teasing the Clitoris

She is tingling all over. Her pussy wants to be touched, but first he takes her to the bathroom so that she can pee before he rubs her there, as he does not want her to have to pee in the middle of his rubbing. He brings her back to the bed, and they have a bite of chocolate and a few raspberries.

She lies down on the bed, perpendicular to him. He sits with his back against some pillows that rest against the headboard. He is right-handed, so his right leg is over her belly and his left leg is under her legs. He spreads her legs, placing her right (outside) leg on a pillow. He goes back to her thighs and starts teasing them with a light touch. He teases her pubic hair, also with a light touch. He lightly touches the outside of her anus with his finger. She is tingling again.

He then tells her that he is going to spread her lips and brush back her pubic hair so that he can better see her clitoris and genitals. He describes how pink and beautiful her clitoris looks to him. Her clitoris is starting to peek out from under her hood. He reports any contractions or color changes that he notices.

He then gets some lubricant and, starting from her perineum, lubricates with moderate to light pressure all over her pussy, except her clitoris. He then strokes up her introitus till he almost gets to her clitoris and then strokes back down. He plays with her inner lips, making sure that they are well lubricated, and tells her how silky and smooth they are. She can hardly wait any longer for her clitoris to be touched.

## Clitoral Stimulation

He lets her know that her wait is almost over. With a strong but friendly grip, he places his left hand with two fingers under each buttock and his thumb resting at the base of her introitus. He then puts a little lubricant on his right index finger (the middle finger is better for some people). He places his right thumb against the shaft of her clitoris, pulling up her hood and exposing the head of her clitoris. He lets her know how shiny and pretty her clitoris is.

He then places his lubricated index finger directly on the upper left quadrant of her clitoris and begins stroking with a light to medium pressure, fairly quickly, using a very short stroke. He lets her know that her clitoris is engorging and that her lips are getting redder and also engorging. He tells her how good it feels to his hand. He can feel contractions with his left thumb, but continues to rub with the same stroke as long as she is going up.

Just before he feels that she won't go higher with the next stroke, he takes a short break. He then goes back to the same stroke and takes her up and up and up, and then takes another break. Her clitoris is now fully engorged, bulbous and beautiful, and he tells her so. He now touches her on different parts of her clitoris, using a consistent stroke. She goes up and up and up, and then he takes a break. He goes back to her favorite spot and takes her up and up and up. He gives her a sip from her glass with the straw.

He brings her down a little with some long strokes and then back up with short, quick ones. She is having abdominal ridging and strong contractions. He reports that to her and tells her that her clitoris is even larger and harder. He keeps peaking her, taking her up and up and either stopping for a break or bringing her down a little with his intention, so that he can bring her up again and again.

She has by now sucked his thumb into her vagina, and he presses down at the base. Nerves from her anus are nearby, and these add to her feeling. He continues to stroke her with his finger on her clitoris. He puts two fingers of his left hand up and under her pubic bone, where the roots of her clitoris are, and slowly, using some pressure, moves them in and out as he continues to rub her clitoris from the top. She feels surrounded and is moaning deeply with pleasure. He does some slow, short strokes on her clitoris that continue to take her up.

He moves his two left fingers to the pocket on the left wall of her vagina as he speeds up the short stroke and takes her even higher. Up and up and up, up and up and up. She says, "Don't stop, don't stop!" and he stops and asks her, "Who do you think is in charge here?" With his left pinkie, he plays with her anus. He brings her up one more time, and this time he says he won't stop, he will take her over, but then he says, "Maybe one more peak," stops for a split second, and then starts again. He does this a number of times as she goes higher and higher, higher than she has ever been. He lets her know that he is there with her, tells her to keep feeling, and he takes her up one more time; this time, he continues to rub.

## Coming Down

She is still at the top of her orgasm, and her contractions are strong as he continues to rub, slowing down his stroke and lightening it but continuing to stroke as she comes down. He strokes more and more slowly as she releases all that energy. He continues as long as there is sensation, using a slow stroke.

He then places his hand over her pubic bone and presses down. He does a pull-up, inserting the two middle fingers of his right hand and pulling up under her pubic bone as he presses his palm down against its top. She is still having contractions, and he presses for a while. He then removes his hand, picks up a washcloth, and firmly removes all the lubricant from her genitals. She has some more contractions as he moves it past her lips and clitoris.

If he is turned on and hard, this is a great time to have intercourse. But she may be so full that all she wants is to lie there and cuddle. She might want to eat some of the delicious food and come down even more. Whatever they decide, this has been one of the best days of her life, and his too.

This is only an example, and as we wrote earlier, we don't expect you to go through all of this every time you make out. Some people may never go through all of this, and that is also fine. Learn what your partner likes by putting attention on them, and then touch them so it pleasures you. Don't get into the "success" mode and continue to rub past the point that she has feeling. Remember, it's better to peak too early than to peak too late.

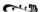

# Love Is Like

Steve wrote this poem for Vera, and we wanted to share it with our readers.

You will be my princess,
And I will be your prince.
I loved you when I met you,
I have loved you ever since.

Love is like a flower,
You water it each day,
Breathe its scented beauty,
Before it goes away.

Love is like a parachute,
It unwinds what once was wound.
It sails along the windstream,
Takes you safely back to ground.

Love is like a fish,
It moves quickly through the sea.
When you think you've caught it,
You have merely set it free.

Love is like a star,
It shines upon your heart.
It can make your night sparkle,
And lighten what is dark.

Love is like a bird,
It appears from high above.
It soars with wing and song,
From its heart it sings of love.

Love is like a tree,
It produces fruit that's sweet.
Creates fresh air to breathe,
And shades you from the heat.

Love is like a fountain,
Shooting bubbles in the air.
Teasing those around her,
With spirit and with flair.

Love is like a rainbow,
It makes you shout, 'hooray!'
When you go to grab it,
Again it moves away.

Love can be magnetic,
Love can go away.
Love can be prophetic,
Love can also stay.

Love can be so sweet,
Love can be profound.
Love can come with heat,
Love can make your heart pound.

Love can be so powerful,
Or a feather in the breeze.
Giving life its meaning,
While keeping things at ease.

Woman, you are so lovable,
Your smell, your skin, your smile,
Blessed are your feelings,
You make everything worthwhile.

Love can be eternal,
One may not apprehend.
A Now that is immortal,
The relationship is friend.

# *Endnotes*

1  See Tor Norretranders, *The User Illusion: Cutting Consciousness Down to Size* (New York, NY: Viking, 1998), p. 127.

2  See Marvin Minsky, *The Society of Mind.* (New York, NY: Simon & Schuster, 1986), p.151.

3  See Eric Haseltine, "Brainworks: Do You See This?" in *Discover Magazine* (October 1999), p.120.

4  See Norretranders, p.210.

5  See Minsky, p.238. Minsky says, "Much of ordinary thought is based on rec-ognizing differences. This is because it is generally useless to do anything that has no discernible effect. To ask if something is significant is virtually to ask, 'What difference does it make?'" Indeed, whenever we talk about cause and effect we're referring to imaginary links that connect the differences we sense. What, indeed, are goals themselves, but ways in which we represent the kinds of changes we might like to make?"

6  See Marvin Harris, *Our Kind: Who We Are, Where We Are, and Where We Are Going: The Evolution of Human Life and Culture* (New York, NY: Harper & Row, 1989), p.330, and Leonard Shlain, *The Alphabet versus the Goddess: The Conflict Between Word and Image* (New York, NY: Penguin Putnam, 1998). Shlain believes that women's second-class status resulted from the introduc-tion of the alphabet and written word and the spread of literacy.

7  See David Simon, *Vital Energy* (New York, NY: John Wiley & Sons, 2000), p.140.

8  See Jared Diamond, *The Third Chimpanzee: The Evolution and Future of the Human Animal* (New York, NY: HarperCollins, 1992), p.195.

9  See Natalie Angier, *Woman: An Intimate Geography* (New York, NY: Houghton Mifflin, 1999), p.63.

10  See Kermit E. Krantz, "Corpus Clitoridis," in *The Classic Clitoris*, Thomas P. Lowry, ed. (Chicago, IL: Nelson Hall, 1978), p.112; originally published in *Obstetrics and Gynecology* 12 (1958): 382–396.

11  See Angier, p.64.

12  See Krantz's discussion of innervation of the human vulva and vagina.

13  See Krantz, and also see Ludwig George Kobelt, "The Female Sex Organs in Humans and Some Mammals," in *The Classic Clitoris*, Thomas P. Lowry, ed. (Chicago, IL: Nelson Hall, 1978), p.19. Originally published in 1844.

14  Other books that aren't entirely devoted to the clitoris, however, are available. Angier's book contains the most useful information on the clitoris that we've found; see pp.62–89.

15  There are other theories about this spot, too: see Angier, p.82.

16  See Krantz, p.111.

17  See Mary Jane Sherfey, *The Nature and Evolution of Female Sexuality* (New York, NY: Random House, 1966), p.85.

18  See Diamond, p.174. He describes experiments in which bowerbird eggs were moved from one region to another. Hatchlings learned nest-building rules by watching older birds.

19  See George B. Schaller, *The Last Panda* (Chicago, IL: University of Chicago Press, 1993), pp.66–69, 71–73.

20 See Angier, p.226, who has some excellent information on this topic.

21 See Richard Dawkins' *Unweaving the Rainbow: Science, Delusion, and the Appetite for Wonder* (New York, NY: Houghton Mifflin Co., 1998), pp.286-313, for an excellent description of the increase in size and capacity of human brains and skulls.

22 See Frans de Waal, *Bonobo: The Forgotten Ape* (Berkeley, CA: University of California Press, 1997.), pp.76–78.

23 See Angier, p.213.

24 See Diamond, p.72.

# Bibliography

Angier, Natalie. *Woman: An Intimate Geography.* New York, NY: Houghton Mifflin, 1999.

Baranco, Vic. *Things I've Heard Vic Say.* Vol. 6. California: More University Press, 1991.

Dawkins, Richard. *Climbing Mount Improbable.* New York, NY: W. W. Norton, 1996.

———. *The Selfish Gene.* Oxford, UK: Oxford University Press, 1976.

———. *Unweaving the Rainbow: Science, Delusion, and the Appetite for Wonder.* New York, NY: Houghton Mifflin Co., 1998.

Diamond, Jared. *Guns, Germs, and Steel: The Fate of Human Societies.* New York, NY: W. W. Norton, 1997.

———. *The Third Chimpanzee: The Evolution and Future of the Human Animal.* New York, NY: HarperCollins, 1992.

Fisher, Helen E. *Anatomy of Love: A Natural History of Monogamy, Adultery, and Divorce.* New York, NY: W. W. Norton, 1992.

———. *The First Sex: The Natural Talents of Women and How They Will Change the World.* New York, NY: Random House, 1999.

———. *The Sex Contract: The Evolution of Human Behavior.* New York, NY: William Morrow, 1982.

Harris, Marvin. *Our Kind: Who We Are, Where We Are, and Where We Are Going: The Evolution of Human Life and Culture.* New York, NY: Harper & Row, 1989.

Harrison, Steven. *Doing Nothing: Coming to the End of the Spiritual Search.* New York, NY: Penguin Putnam, 1997.

Haseltine, Eric. "Brainworks: Do You See This?" *Discover Magazine,* October 1999.

Kinsey, Alfred, Paul H. Gebhard, Clyde E. Martin, and Wardell B. Pomeroy. *Sexual Behavior in the Human Female.* Philadelphia, PA: W. B. Saunders Company, 1953.

Lowry, Thomas P., ed. *The Classic Clitoris.* Chicago, IL: Nelson Hall, 1978. Includes "Corpus Clitoridis," by Kermit E. Krantz, about clitoral anatomy, and "The Female Sex Organs in Humans and Some Mammals," by Ludwig George Kobelt, a description of the clitoris. Krantz's article was originally published in *Obstetrics and Gynecology* 12 (1958): 382-396. Kobelt's article was first published in 1844.

Margulis, Lynn, and Dorion Sagan. *What Is Sex?* New York, NY: Simon & Schuster, 1997.

Masters, William H., Virginia E. Johnson, and Robert C. Kolodny. *Sex and Human Loving.* Boston, MA: Little, Brown and Co., 1982.

Minsky, Marvin. *The Society of Mind.* New York, NY: Simon & Schuster, 1986.

Norretranders, Tor. *The User Illusion: Cutting Consciousness Down to Size.* New York, NY: Viking, 1998.

Schaller, George B. *The Last Panda.* Chicago, IL: University of Chicago Press, 1993.

Sherfey, Mary Jane. *The Nature and Evolution of Female Sexuality.* New York, NY: Random House, 1966.

Shlain, Leonard. *The Alphabet versus the Goddess: The Conflict Between Word and Image.* New York, NY: Penguin Putnam, 1998.

Simon, David. *Vital Energy.* New York, NY: John Wiley & Sons, 2000.

Taylor, Patricia H. *The Enchantment of Opposites: How to Create Great Relationships.* Oakland, CA: Traveling Artists Press, 1997.

Waal, Frans de. "Bonobo: Sex and Society," *Scientific American,* March 1995.

———. *Bonobo: The Forgotten Ape.* Berkeley, CA: University of California Press, 1997.

Wilber, Ken. *A Brief History of Everything.* Boston, MA: Shambhala Publications, Inc., 1996.

———. *Marriage of Sense and Soul: Integrating Science and Religion.* New York, NY: Random House, 1998.

Woods, Margo. *Tantra and Self Love.* San Diego, CA: Omphaloskepsis Press, 1981.

# Index

## A

abdominal ridging, 98

Abolene, 83

acquired immune deficiency syndrome
(AIDS), 163, 164

active roles, 29, 31

anger, 39–40, 44–45

Angier, Natalie, 149, 154

anus, 52, 91

apex, penis, 57, 91

appreciation, 42

approval, 38–39

Astroglide, 83

attention, and seduction, 4

attractiveness, 43, 174

## B

beauty, 43

begging, 133–134

bonobos, 153–155; bonobo position, 139

## C

candidiasis, 165

cause and effect, 30–33

cervix, 88

change, resistance to, 15

chimpanzees, 153–155

chlamydia, 165

clitorial hood, 52, 53, 173

clitoris, 24, 50–55; anchoring, 84; role of,
4; sensitivity, 173

coercion, 129

communication, 40–43, 102–120, 175, 185

compliments, 75

condoms, 164

connections (exercise), 64–65

consciousness, and orgasm, 11–15

consent, 5

contractions, vaginal, 98

control, giving up, 116

crura, 54

cunnilingus, 78, 184

cycles, synchronous, 147

## D

dancing on the clitoris (technique), 128

Dawkins, Richard, 48

dental dams, 164

detumescing, 99–100

DNA exchange, 20

"doing," definition, 30, 31

## E

effect, 30–33

ejaculation, preventing, 91; premature,
180

ejaculatory fluid, 98

emotions, 17–18

engorgement, clitoral, 51–54; female, 24;
male, 88

205

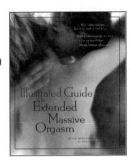
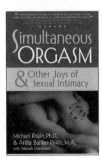

# SEXUAL SELF-HELP FOR EVERYONE
## Three books *by* Barbara Keesling, Ph.D.

### SEXUAL PLEASURE: Reaching New Heights of Sexual Arousal and Intimacy

This book is for anyone who wants to make love without anxiety or pressure, which starts with learning to enjoy touching and being touched. It shows you how to focus on your desire, which puts you in touch with your body and leads to pleasure for both partners.

*Sexual Pleasure* introduces readers to the unique **sensate focus** exercises, to be done alone and with a partner, to increase sensual awareness. The exercises are independent of sexual orientation and can be used by those who have physical limitations, those who are learning about sexuality—anyone interested in better sex.

*224 pages ... 14 b/w photos ... Paperback $14.95*

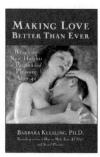

### MAKING LOVE BETTER THAN EVER: Reaching New Heights of Passion and Pleasure After 40

Great sex is not reserved for those under 40. With maturity comes the potential for a multi-faceted loving that draws from all we are and deepens our ties. This is the loving that sustains relationships into later years.

In this book, Dr. Keesling shows couples how to reignite sexual feelings and reconnect emotionally. She provides body-image and caress exercises that heighten sexual response and expand sexual potential, build self-esteem, open the lines of communication, and promote playfulness, spontaneity, and joy.

*208 pages ... 14 b/w photos ... Paperback $13.95*

### Rx SEX: Making Love Is the Best Medicine

This book offers rare information about the healing powers of sex. *Rx Sex* asks what you want to heal—emotions, physical problems, or a relationship—and directs you to a setting and exercises that are right for you. The health benefits of making love include:

\*\* strengthening your immune system, breathing and circulation; healthier skin, hair and eyes; pain relief

\*\* relieving depression and anxiety; improving concentration and memory; restoring a positive body image

*192 pages ... 14 b/w photos ... Paperback $13.95*

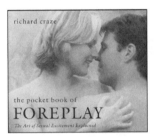
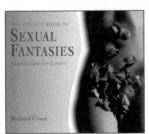

# ORDER FORM

10% DISCOUNT on orders of $50 or more —
20% DISCOUNT on orders of $150 or more —
30% DISCOUNT on orders of $500 or more —
*On cost of books for fully prepaid orders*

NAME

ADDRESS

CITY/STATE                                    ZIP/POSTCODE

PHONE                                         COUNTRY (outside of U.S.)

| TITLE | QTY | PRICE | TOTAL |
|---|---|---|---|
| Extended Massive Orgasm (paperback) | | @ $ 14.95 | |
| The Illustrated Guide to EMO (paperback) | | @ $ 16.95 | |

*Prices subject to change without notice*

*Please list other titles below:*

| | | |
|---|---|---|
| | @ $ | |
| | @ $ | |
| | @ $ | |
| | @ $ | |
| | @ $ | |
| | @ $ | |
| | @ $ | |

*Check here to receive our book catalog* ❏        *FREE*

**Shipping Costs**

*By Priority Mail: first book $4.50, each additional book $1.00*
*By UPS and to Canada: first book $5.50, each additional book $1.50*
*For rush orders and other countries call us at (510) 865-5282*

| | |
|---|---|
| TOTAL | _____ |
| Less discount @_____% | (_____) |
| TOTAL COST OF BOOKS | _____ |
| Calif. residents add sales tax | _____ |
| Shipping & handling | _____ |
| **TOTAL ENCLOSED** | _____ |

*Please pay in U.S. funds only*

❏ Check ❏ Money Order ❏ Visa ❏ Mastercard ❏ Discover

Card #_____ Exp. date_____

Signature_____

*Complete and mail to:*
**Hunter House Inc., Publishers**
PO Box 2914, Alameda CA 94501-0914
**Website: www.hunterhouse.com**
Orders: (800) 266-5592 or email: ordering@hunterhouse.com
Phone (510) 865-5282 Fax (510) 865-4295

EMO-R3 7/2002